# THE
# HOT BODY
# DIET

THE PLAN TO
**RADICALLY TRANSFORM**
YOUR BODY
IN **28 DAYS**

# MICHELLE LEWIN

with DR. SAMAR YORDE

CELEBRA
NEW YORK

CELEBRA
Published by Berkley
An imprint of Penguin Random House LLC
375 Hudson Street, New York, New York 10014

Library of Congress Cataloging-in-Publication Data

Names: Lewin, Michelle, author. | Yorde, Samar, author.
Title: The hot body diet: the plan to radically transform your body in 28
days/Michelle Lewin with Dr. Samar Yorde.
Description: First edition. | New York: Celebra, 2018.
Identifiers: LCCN 2017061333| ISBN 9780399585449 (paperback) |
ISBN 9780399585555 (e-book)
Subjects: LCSH: Weight loss. | Exercise. | Nutrition. | BISAC: HEALTH &
FITNESS/Diets. | HEALTH & FITNESS/Nutrition. | HEALTH & FITNESS/
Weight Loss.
Classification: LCC RM222.2.L4456 2018 | DDC 613.2/5—dc23
LC record available at https://lccn.loc.gov/2017061333

First Edition: June 2018

Printed in the United States of America
1   3   5   7   9   10   8   6   4   2

Cover art by LHGFX Photography
Cover design by Katie Anderson
Book design by Pauline Neuwrith

*For God, who allows me to be in this world doing what I love.*

*For my mom, who gave me life and the strength
to achieve whatever I set out to do.*

*For Jimmy, who guides me, accompanies me,
and always pushes me forward.*

*For everyone who follows me on social media,
because your caring and enthusiasm
motivate me to become my best self.*

# CONTENTS

# FOREWORD

**L**ife will never cease to amaze us. God puts in our path people and situations that come to improve our life for good, even if we don't necessarily realize it in the moment. There are things that happen when we least expect them, that shake us up and change our way of thinking and radically transform our lives. Both Michelle Lewin and I are a testament to this, in two very different ways.

I am a doctor, a specialist in public health and obesity medicine. In the United States I studied to become a health coach, speaker, writer, and lecturer. In my career I've had the opportunity to see hundreds of patients suffering from obesity as well as a number of diseases associated with being overweight. As a doctor I understand that obesity is a weapon of mass destruction, an epidemic that we must tackle. That's why over the past six years I have been on a path toward education and prevention through my @soysaludable social networking account.

Through this multimedia platform, I've managed to motivate and change the lives of thousands of people, inspiring them to eat well, achieve a healthy weight, exercise regularly, and overcome their mental barriers. While I was teaching others how to eat healthily and adopt healthy lifestyle habits, I continued to treat patients through in-person and online consultations. The result was almost always the same: my patients achieved impressive changes both in their weight and in their lifestyle.

Yet even though it's hard to believe, in spite of having helped so many people through my advice on health and nutrition, I myself wasn't able to make my own radical change in order to shed my extra pounds and gain control over the anxiety that stymied my efforts. It was a living nightmare: the doctor who helped others lose weight was unable to achieve her own weight goals and gain control over her metabolism and hormones. Something was terribly wrong and I myself couldn't even believe it.

I come from the world of obesity, which started to take over my life, little by little, after I had my first child. At a certain point I weighed over 220 pounds, which had terrible consequences for my self-esteem and physical health. It was just around that time that I decided to specialize in obesity medicine in the hopes of saving myself from this terrible condition. With great effort, and over the course of several years, I managed to lose about forty pounds, but then I fell into a zone of resistance, where I was able to lose a few pounds only to gain them back again. Over time, my weight-loss journey stalled completely, and just like many of the women reading this book, I was eager to solve my problem forever.

Two years ago I left Venezuela and moved to Miami, where I met Michelle and gave her my first book of healthy recipes. I discovered Michelle through social media and I was struck by her transformation. Yes, I say transformation, because Michelle wasn't born with that body we all admire so much. Not at all. Her body is the product of much effort, discipline, and sacrifice. From the moment I met her, I was delighted with her humbleness and good energy, and I can say that we became friends on day one. Then I met her husband, Jimmy, a fitness fanatic with an impressive sense of humor and a creative mind that never stops. Jimmy and Michelle are a delightful couple and together they have dedicated their lives to promoting fitness and a healthy lifestyle throughout the world.

On a couple of occasions over the course of the past two years, Michelle and Jimmy motivated me to lose the weight I needed to lose in order to reach my goal. They gave me advice and even invited me to train with them, but I was still too focused on anything—work, anxiety, money, relationships, wanting to feel more secure—other than my transformation. I had forty pounds to lose and was overwhelmed with anxiety over the situations I had had to face after leaving Venezuela to start a new life in the United States. My mind was a factory of silly fears and excuses.

One day, Jimmy and Michelle said to me, "Let's make it a public challenge. We'll help you lose weight: you'll train with Michelle and follow a diet plan." The idea terrified me, but I decided to run with it. In the first forty-five days, I managed to lose almost fourteen pounds. I was elated and clung to the motivation they so generously gave me. Then Michelle and Jimmy went away for a long time, and I was left alone, without the sufficient willpower to stay on track. My weight loss stalled and the following month, when Christmas came around, I even managed to gain a few pounds. Over the following months, I felt depressed because I hate to fail. And on top of that, I also felt like I was letting my two mentors down. I felt awful.

I was full of doubts and regrets, until one day Michelle, with that sweet and tough tone of hers, confronted me with my deepest fears, saying, "The thing is, you don't really want to do it, because if you did, you would have already done it. You always accomplish what you set your mind to, but this is something you don't really want." Her words were like a bucket of cold water.

And then life, or God, or whatever you want to call it made its move.

A few years ago, Michelle and I put together a healthy-recipe book and we were looking for a publisher. We ended up finding a home at Penguin Random House, where a team of visionaries and enthusiasts was willing to share Michelle's eating, training, and motivation secrets with the rest of the world. In the end, we decided to save that cookbook for a second book and to start with a book about Michelle's life, her food secrets, and her meal plan to achieve a fabulous, strong, and healthy body.

Michelle, who is a woman of few words but great actions and results, who was already planning on sharing her meal plan and recipes with her entire community of followers, accepted the offer, but not before asking me to support her as a doctor and writer, in the adventure of putting together this book. I was delighted with the idea: who better than Michelle to motivate an entire community of women who dream of getting beyond what they could have imagined? It was my own dream to work with her in writing and putting together this book, let alone reading it from beginning to end.

So Michelle and I started to write this book together, and we developed recipes based on her eating style. As we wrote, I began to apply everything I learned from her to my own life. It was simple: I had the knowledge, the experience, and the perfect motivation to do it—the decision to write this book was like dropping an atomic bomb on my entire past in order to start a new life, doing things right.

Sure enough, I started to see the changes, and the extra pounds began to melt away. Doing what Michelle does—learning how to eat, train, supplement, and motivate myself—inspired me and, even more, enriched the lives of the people who follow me as well as my own life. It seemed magical to be able to compile Michelle's experience in a book, with all the scientific knowledge I had accumulated through my research as a doctor. And so we began the process, which lasted just over six months, of collecting the information. We spent many long hours together in conversation. I thoroughly recorded everything we discussed, and then I would go back and look for the scientific evidence to support her experience and knowledge.

The day I met Michelle, I didn't think she would change my life. And she changed it for good.

Before, I was a woman of much knowledge but little action. Now I understand that without action, there are no results. Today, at age forty-seven and a grandmother, I can humbly say that I feel better than ever. I've managed to get closer to the body of my dreams thanks to the Hot Body Diet. Not only was I able to get rid of the extra pounds; I gained a universe in self-esteem, energy, enthusiasm, and the desire to help others change their lives.

Today you have in your hands a book that contains Michelle's experience, enriched by the most current advances in medicine, nutrition, and metabolic study. Here you will learn about motivation, good habits, nutrition, hormones, metabolic control, supplements, vitamins, and healthy recipes. It's all you need to know to rebuild your body or take it to its maximum potential of beauty and well-being.

I can say that this will be one of the most honest and complete books you will ever read. Michelle didn't learn by studying; she learned by doing, practicing, failing, and starting up again—over and over. Hers is a process of trial and error, one with striking results that speak for themselves. And that's worth more than anything you'll ever read on the Internet or at the library. Because a single day of action is worth so much more than a month spent reading or having good intentions.

I want you to take this book very seriously. I want you to read each chapter, multiple times if necessary. Because in the end, when you stand with your arms high in the circle of winners, light as a feather and strong as a lioness, you will experience the immense joy of having conquered your mind and your body and connected with the most wonderful force there is: the will to overcome adversity and to overcome yourself. You will see that every drop of sweat, every meal, every day lived will have been worth it.

This book will make you feel fabulous: physically strong and mentally indestructible. It will be your plan to win, once and for all, the war against your fears and the excess weight you have been carrying for all these years. Here is your road map to victory. You will thank God every day for having it, just as I thanked him for putting it in my path.

May good things come your way; this is just the beginning! And to you, Michelle: I will always thank you for touching my life.

Dr. Samar Yorde
@SoySaludable

# INTRODUCTION

**H**i! **I'm Michelle** Lewin, a girl like you who one day discovered a great passion that changed her life: fitness. I also discovered a method of training and eating that has allowed me to achieve incredible results, travel the world, and become a sports model known to millions of people around the world.

You might already know me from social media, or perhaps you've seen my pictures and videos in magazines or on the Internet. Or this might be the very first time you have come in contact with me. But regardless of whether you know me or not, you probably don't know my story, the one that brought me to where I am today, the one I want to share with you.

I am no fairy-tale princess, nor have I had a perfect life. I am a woman who has learned to overcome life's challenges. And I have encountered quite a few. Nothing in my life has been easy or free. I have dedicated the past few years of my life to fitness. My ultimate goal is—and will continue to be—to maintain a naturally thin, feminine, harmonious, strong, attractive, and healthy body that will allow me to feel good about myself and inspire and motivate millions of women to do the same. It is also very important for me to keep a calm, disciplined, and determined mind in order never to abandon this path. I like to share my workout routines with my followers, and I like it even more when I hear their stories at events or see their wonderful results in photos.

I decided to write this book because over the past three years, many women have asked me about the eating plan I follow in order to achieve the body that everyone sees on social media. I have so much to say and share that, instead of publishing advice and tips as isolated tidbits that might get lost on my social media timelines, I decided to compile everything I've learned in this complete guide that you can use to achieve your goals.

I want to push you to make the decision to change everything you don't like about your body, to reach the best version of yourself and become the fabulous woman you've always dreamed of becoming. I want to support you in the same way Jimmy Lewin—my husband, accomplice, manager, and main motivator—has supported me. He is the man who changed my life for the better.

In this book you'll find all the information you need, and I can guarantee that if you do what I say and you commit to following my advice with honesty and generosity, you'll go farther than you've ever imagined. Just like me. My results speak for themselves.

The first thing I have to tell you—and I know that deep down you already know this—is that there is no diet or eating plan that works the same way for everyone. There are many factors that determine how many calories you need to consume to achieve your goals, and the first thing you need to decide is what you want to accomplish. A diet plan for weight loss isn't the same as one designed to gain a more toned physique or to increase muscle mass. Nor should a small, 4'11", sedentary woman eat the same amount of food as a 5'10" athlete, for example. There are other important factors, such as age, metabolism, muscle mass, starting weight, bone structure, living conditions, hormonal health, basic diseases, and so on.

I am not a nutritionist or a health coach (and I don't pretend to be one), but my body is the result of the experience I've accumulated over years of doing what works for me and staying away from what sets me off track. As Tony Robbins, the number one motivational speaker in the world, would say, "I have a PhD in RESULTS." Consider me a very experienced friend who is happy and proud of her results and wants you to feel the same.

With regards to scientific evidence upon which this book is based, I complemented my experience with the knowledge of Dr. Samar Yorde, a doctor and health coach who is passionate about life and healthy cooking. She brought scientific data, recipes, and many other valuable contributions to this book. The two of us have worked on putting together a complete book in which I explain everything you need to know to achieve quick results that are both effective and healthy. And that's the magic of this book: by the time you reach the end, you will have all my experience, methods, and results, supported and validated by the scientific evidence provided by an expert—because my number one priority is that you do things the right way.

This is the most honest book you will ever read. There's no cheap advertising here and there won't be any magic transformations if you're not willing to put in the effort. Here you will understand that to achieve extraordinary results, you have to push yourself. A lot. I have learned everything I know from the effort, the commitment, and the techniques of those who have guided and supported me along the way.

## SOME THINGS MONEY CAN'T BUY

My own body is the lab where I have tested this exercise-and-meal plan. I know what works and what doesn't, and I would go so far as to say that I can manipulate my body to my liking. I know exactly what I need to eat for a competition or a photo shoot, and when I can afford to eat a giant hamburger with fries without feeling guilty or affecting my muscle definition. I don't torture myself by going on extreme diets, nor am I obsessed; I just learned to eat in a natural and balanced way to get the energy I need for my body to function in the best way possible and become a fat-burning machine.

I am living the life I worked for, one I earned by sacrificing ice cream and parties, one I sweated for every time I pushed myself to the max, facing that last repetition, that extra weight, fighting the temptation to stay in bed when all I wanted was one more hour of sleep but simply had to get up. I have a body built on effort, not instant gratification, the operating room, or the silly idea that "money buys you everything."

The average person may not notice the difference between abs made in an operating room and abs that are the product of training and a balanced diet. But there's a difference. I can spot it immediately. Operating-room abs may seem real at first, but once you look closely you can see the difference. Because the fact is, if someone has a body-fat percentage so low that you can spot a six-pack, the rest of the body is usually just as toned. And in the case of fake abs, it isn't. People who turn to magical solutions (such as injecting harmful substances into their buttocks or getting a fake six-pack, for example) aren't only putting their health at risk; they're really fooling only themselves.

In this book I want to share with you the postcards of a trip that I embarked on a few years ago and that has taken me to visit a wide variety of kitchens, gyms, restaurants, cities, and emotions. We can take this trip together, enjoying life, eating healthily, finding a thousand good reasons to select the right foods, do your cardio, lift that last weight, and finish those last reps even though they make you want to scream.

I want to inspire you to believe that anything is possible, that you can change your mind and body, that you can overcome your weaknesses and become your best self. Because anything is possible as long as you want it and decide it.

One day someone I love very much told me that I shouldn't compete in fitness, that it wasn't for me, that I didn't have the strength or the desire to do it. I will tell you this story later, but for now I can say that at that moment I went mad with indignation. But my tears turned into fuel for a fire that was already burning in my heart. The result? I am a fire, a volcano in flames, and when someone tells me there's something I "can't do," I find strength I didn't even know I had in order to do it. Thanks to those tough but well-intended—or shall I say perfect—words, I was able to make a radical change and transform my body from ordinary to extraordinary in just four weeks.

Over the course of those twenty-eight days of intense training and mindful eating, I changed my body in such a way that I went from coming in last place at my first fitness competition to coming in second among a group of one hundred top-tier competitors. After that I repeated the plan for another twenty-eight days and the following month I managed to win first place overall at the 2013 Tampa Bay Pro Show, one of the most prestigious and credible fitness events in the United States.

That's why I designed this twenty-eight-day plan for you: because if I was able to radically change my body in just twenty-eight days, you can do it too. And you might not reach your final goal in twenty-eight days, but that first change will give you the motivation to repeat the cycle until you achieve it.

## NO ONE SAID IT WOULD BE EASY

I know from experience that it's hard to make drastic changes, and if you come from eating hamburgers and pizza every day, you will probably start to lose weight by making just a few small changes and replacements. But you probably won't get much further, because in order to achieve radical changes in your body you have to make radical changes to your lifestyle. Unless you want to make just a slight improvement and aren't willing to take it to the next level, this is nonnegotiable. In the end it's your decision and yours only.

I'm not going to trick you by telling you that you can eat whatever you want, in small amounts, and achieve a toned body in just a few months. Nor will I tell you that you can eat as much food as you want as long as it's healthy food, because you won't get anywhere doing that either. And I will definitely not tell you to add all sorts of sauces and processed foods to your "healthy" preparations, because if you do you will most certainly fail before you even begin.

What you eat is very important, but how you eat it is even more important. The macronutrients (carbohydrates, proteins, and fats), vitamins, and minerals you select; the amounts or portions you eat; the times at which you eat them; how you prepare them; the relationship between what you eat and the exercise you do and even supplements you take . . . all play a fundamental role in how and when you achieve your goals.

I designed this diet plan for you, because I have tried it on myself and it has allowed me to win competitions and get contracts as a fitness model, and most importantly, it has allowed me to overcome my own weaknesses, gain self-esteem, and feel like I've never felt before. If it worked for me, it will work for you too, and you deserve to have the body and the life you want. Just ask yourself: how strong is my passion, and what's really motivating me to change my body? This is where you need to start.

## A GIFT FOR YOU

In order to thank you, my friends and followers, for all the love and support you have given me through social media, I want to share with you a diet plan that really does work, along with a few simple recipes I love because they are delicious and I can enjoy them without guilt, without excesses, without losing—over the course of a couple of meals—what has cost months of hard training to earn.

I'm not going to give you a strict diet plan, because that's not how we eat in real life. I will share my ideal meal plan for twenty-eight days, adapted to three lifestyles (sedentary, active, athlete), with so many options to vary your meals that you can repeat it without getting bored, until you reach your final goal.

I hope that you like this plan and that you can adapt it to your life. But before you begin, remember that no advice shared in this book can replace the advice of a health professional. I want to share what has worked for me: my secret formula for looking good and, above all, feeling powerful. I encourage you to apply it to your own life so you can get to where you never imagined, regardless of your age or current weight.

No matter how you look today, what matters most is who you will become. And remember, be patient! It's about moving forward one day at a time. And once you arrive at your destination, nothing and no one can stop that internal force—it will far surpass the strength of your muscles!

Welcome to my world. Today is the day you start to become your best self! And I will be by your side throughout this entire journey so we can celebrate your achievements together. Let's go! I want to see your changes, and share them with the world. This is just the beginning!

Michelle Lewin

# THE
# HOT BODY
# DIET

# 1.

# WHERE I COME FROM

I am not a fairy-tale princess, nor have I led a charmed life. My story is one of struggle, dedication, and discipline to overcome my own barriers and reach where I am today. I still have a way to go, but I will always take on new challenges. I am in love with this life that I decided to build, and it has motivated me to help other women overcome their own barriers in order to become their best selves. I will give you my secret formula to discover your personal strength, change your life habits, break down every single one of your barriers, and achieve a strong and healthy body. Because if I was able to do it, so can you. And if you can't, it's just because you don't want to. Period.

—MICHELLE LEWIN

**Y**ou've probably seen my pictures on social media, where I'm almost always posing in a swimsuit or sportswear. Or you may have learned some of the exercise routines I've shared online. You may have also followed my travels and fun times through Instagram stories or Snapchat. Perhaps you've already downloaded my workouts at https://www.fitplan app.com/athletes/michelle-lewin, or you're training with my platform at www.lewinfitnessplatform.com and you feel connected and even inspired by the training program I've designed for you. You probably feel like you and I are close, but the truth is, you don't really know me yet. That's why I want to tell you where I come from and, most of all, how I came to you.

Some people are born in perfect homes and their lives are filled with blessings. Others may not have experienced the joy of coming to the world in a golden cradle and feeling absolute love and protection through childhood. But a difficult start doesn't necessarily mean that we can't make our dreams come true or that we'll fail to achieve what we want in life. My story made me strong. I thank God for everything I have experienced, because it's what has made me into the woman I am today.

> **The train doesn't arrive just once. It comes through several times, until the day comes when you decide to board it. And as long as you don't, you'll be stuck in the same station, immobile, paralyzed, complaining to God about how unfair your life is.**
>
> **—MICHELLE LEWIN**

As a girl I was always very quiet—shy, even—yet I had a deep desire to change what I didn't like about my life. And allow me to take this opportunity to give you a first piece of advice you should never forget: The moment you've been hoping for will always come, and you will be able to take advantage of it as long as you truly want it and are willing to make a change. When you want something, declare it, work for it, and you will see it come true.

## "ONCE UPON A TIME . . ."

That's how I would have wanted my story to start. I wanted it to start like one of the children's books I loved so much when I was little. I was the girl who dreamed of being a princess, served, loved, and doted upon by all. The reality was very different: I wasn't a princess, I didn't live in a castle, nor were there many people who made me feel wanted. The most important person in my life was my mother, my greatest protector and my personal heroine.

My mom is my best friend. From Colombia, she is a humble, intelligent woman who had me at just seventeen, an age at which most of us are still very inexperienced and rebellious and are definitely not ready to face such a huge responsibility. Hoping to escape from a tense family situation, she fell in love with a young man from a good family—a helicopter pilot and the son of a member of the Venezuelan military—and dreamed of changing her life. But that was nothing but a dream. My father ignored me from the moment I was conceived and never took responsibility for my mother or for me.

Years later, I learned that when my mom was five or six months pregnant with me, my dad suggested that she not have me, that she "solve that problem," but my mom decided to keep me. I arrived in this world assisted by the Red Cross of the city of Valencia, Venezuela, since my mother didn't have the money to pay for a private clinic. Surviving that possible abortion was my first victory. Thank God my mother decided to save me. And here I am today, telling my story.

I grew up in Maracay, Venezuela, where I lived with my mom and grandmother. I spent the first years of my life in a humble apartment, surrounded by tons of love and protection. When I was eight months old, my mother fell in love with a man named Luigi. His family was Italian and they discriminated against my mother because she was Colombian and a single mother. But Luigi fought his family in order to be with my mother, and he gave me lots of love and support during my early life. Luigi and my mother had two children, Antonieta and Pascual, my beloved siblings and lifelong companions. Antonieta was born when I was four years old, and then two years later came Pascual. Their births changed some things in my relationship with my "dad." At that age I found it a bit difficult to understand why my "Papa Luigi" paid more attention to my siblings—I felt that he preferred them over me, and that made me feel sad and displaced. But thankfully his family loved me very much and they filled my life with loving moments.

Of my real dad I know close to nothing. I grew up knowing that Luigi was not my dad, and even though it hurt that he seemed to prefer my siblings, I had a very happy childhood. Luigi was an excellent father who gave me an education, support, and all the affection a child could ever need.

## "WHEN I WAS FOURTEEN, I GREW UP. . . ."

When I was fourteen years old, my life took a 180-degree turn. My mother decided to divorce my "Papa Luigi," due to irreconcilable differences between herself and his family. After the divorce, Luigi moved in with another woman, but I didn't approve of the relationship and I confronted him about it. My worst mistake was to tell him, in the midst of a childish fit, that he had no right over me because he wasn't my dad. I was jealous and I didn't want to accept that he was with a woman other than my mom. My words hurt him very much, and he replied: "If I'm not your dad, then I won't support you anymore." And he didn't.

At the age of fourteen, I could have never imagined that at that exact moment my "Papa Luigi" was divorcing me too. With the separation I lost his support in every way: he stopped talking to me, paying for my school, buying my clothes and food. I lost my health insurance, and the day I graduated from school my mother still owed several monthly payments. The divorce made my mother very depressed, and she had to go out and find work to support our family. And at that moment, I too began to take on greater responsibilities.

Since my mother wasn't home a lot, I had to take care of the house and my siblings. We fell into a situation of critical poverty, and I managed to survive while my mother struggled to get ahead. We lived in a run-down apartment full of cockroaches where we had no comforts, no food. We often went to bed without dinner, we ate the cheapest food in Venezuela, and we always counted on a generous neighbor to give us something to eat. I wanted to help my mom and get a job but no one was willing to hire me because I was still a minor.

I finally managed to get my first job just before I turned sixteen. It was as a cleaning assistant in a dental office; I had to clean the office and the equipment. Later I worked at a plastic-surgery clinic, then at a hardware store carrying building materials. Later I found work selling cell phones, and then I started working at another clinic . . . I never shied away from any kind of work, because I needed to pay for my education and help support my family. While I was working I was able to finish high school, and I even graduated with a technical degree in business administration and as a flight attendant.

## MOM, WHEN WILL OUR LIVES FINALLY CHANGE?

When I was between the ages of seventeen and twenty-three, one could say that I led a normal life: surviving, studying, and working just like most lower-class girls my age, who needed to work in order to live. I studied hard and worked hard too, but I also went out with friends and enjoyed life. Yet when Christmas and New Year's came around, I was always hit with a bout of nostalgia. Most of the time my mother, my siblings, and I spent Christmas and New Year's in our apartment without much money for gifts or celebrations. We would ring in the New Year in our pajamas, standing on a balcony as we watched our neighbors' fireworks and celebrations, and then we'd go to bed as on every other day of the year. Nothing special. I'll never forget that every year I'd cry and ask my mother, "When will our lives change?" Then, when I was twenty-three and Christmas rolled around, my mother finally said to me: "This year things are going to change. I can feel it."

And they did.

## MY "BEFORE" BODY

Surely you must be wondering what my body looked like back then. Well, I can tell you that I was always very thin, shy, unhappy, and insecure, and I didn't like the way I looked. In fact I didn't like my body at all; I hated my legs because they were too thin, and my self-esteem was at an all-time low. I couldn't stand it when other people looked at me, and I was very nervous. I wanted to be invisible to everyone around me, and I spent many years of my life feeling anxious and asocial. When I was seventeen I started going to the gym thanks to my mom, who was going to the gym to get over her depression. At first I'd go just to keep her company, but soon enough I began to train because I wanted to tone my legs, and little by little I was able to achieve a toned body and legs.

## LIFE CAN CHANGE AT ANY TIME....

When I was twenty-three, my mom took me on a trip with her friends to Isla Margarita in Venezuela, and that trip changed my life. We went over my spring break, and one day when I was lying on the beach a foreigner—burly, athletic, and attractive—came up to me. His Spanish was not perfect, but I remember he asked if he could take a picture of me, and then we exchanged e-mail addresses. That's how we started a long-distance relationship through e-mails and Facebook messages—I could have never imagined that that fortuitous encounter would ultimately bring me to where I am today.

Jimmy was Swedish, and he had been obsessed with fitness and training since the age of eighteen. He was also the manager of a major Swedish tourism operator, which kept him traveling around the world. From time to time he traveled to Isla Margarita, and he would do everything in his power to fly me there so we could spend some time together. Thus began the most beautiful relationship I could have ever imagined. After a while he began to ask me to accompany him on his trips to Europe, while motivating me to continue training. A year later, when we were on a cruise, he asked me to marry him, a request I was delighted to accept since I was very much in love. After we got married we first moved to Italy, then to Spain, and then to Sweden. I loved everything about these experiences, but it wasn't easy for me to adapt to our new life: we clashed often, due to our differences in culture, personality, language, and even in our way of seeing life.

## YES, THERE WERE TIMES WHEN I LET MYSELF GO

When I married Jimmy I was training three times a week and eating anything I wanted (risotto, pizza, burgers, and so on). I never watched what I ate, but I had a genetic tendency to be thin. After we got married we moved to Italy, where I stopped training, continued to eat anything I wanted, and ultimately started gaining weight.

In Italy, I assumed the role of the housewife, the woman who cooks and greets her husband when he comes home from work, and I suddenly ceased to have my own aspirations. I stopped training the way I had before, and I became completely sedentary: all I wanted to do was eat and watch TV. Jimmy felt that I was wasting my time, and I really was wasting it. He worked all day and I did nothing productive other than cooking and taking care of the house. Over the course of our time in Italy, I gained about twenty pounds. There were moments of tension when Jimmy, who was concerned about my attitude, tried to help me control what I ate. I now understand that it was for my own good, but at the time I wanted to kill him. He'd constantly suggest that I go to the gym to work out, and at times I felt as if I was going to suffocate. In Italy I let myself go. Yes, I too have had times when I let myself go.

Jimmy is passionate about the fitness lifestyle, and he became more and more concerned about my defiant attitude and the fact that I was letting myself go. He was an active businessman and my attitude came as a huge shock to him. We had a hard time getting used to each other.

## I COULDN'T BE A MODEL IN SPAIN

After Italy, we moved to Barcelona, Spain, hoping to find better job opportunities for me, a move that only enhanced our differences even more. He wanted to help me in his own way, Swedish style, by restricting my intake of certain foods. In Spain I started to train again, and for the first time in my life I tried to change my eating habits. I had no work permit, and the process of obtaining one took about five months, so in the meantime I had to work handing out flyers on the street. I was trying to make a living and was willing to do any kind of decent work that allowed me to earn a few euros.

In Barcelona I visited several modeling agencies, and they all rejected me—I wasn't thin enough or tall enough to be a model. I am obviously not tall enough to be a runway model, so at one of the agencies I visited someone said to me: "If you want to have a chance at being a model you should move to Miami—that's the place for you, not Spain." I sincerely hope that the person who said that to me buys this book so he can find out how grateful I am that he rejected me and suggested I come to Miami, the place where God wanted my dream to come true.

Since I wasn't able to get a job in Barcelona, Jimmy and I decided to move to Miami. I have to confess that I never saw myself as a model. I had done some modeling work but always on a small scale and nobody really knew me. But Jimmy believed in me more than I believed in myself. He saw potential in me and was determined to take photos and work with photographers, and all I did was follow his lead. He believed in me despite the fact that I didn't have a toned body. Jimmy believed in me to such a degree that he decided to quit his company in order to focus on managing my modeling career in Miami.

## AND SO WE MOVED TO MIAMI. . . .

Jimmy saw me as a star, a diamond in the rough, and in Miami he motivated me to train my body properly, tweak my diet, create consistent training routines, and take the right supplements. He even motivated me to enroll in my first fitness competition. My mom was the first person to get me into a gym, but Jimmy was the one who pushed me to join the challenging, demanding, and competitive world of fitness that I love so much.

In Miami we applied to become US residents but the process wasn't easy. Some friends told me that I might improve my chances if I became a fitness athlete, in addition to my work as a model. And that's when I understood that entering competitions and becoming a fitness athlete would help me become a legal resident of the United States.

I changed my attitude, started taking more of Jimmy's advice, and doing *almost* everything he suggested in order to eat right, train more, and improve my body. At the time I had strong, toned legs but I had never done much work on my upper body. I trained on my own, but I started to prepare as best I could for the competitions I was about to face.

## THE DEFEAT THAT CHANGED MY LIFE . . .

I have always wanted to be the best at whatever challenge I embark on. I hate feeling defeated, but just like everyone else, I have lost. Yet there is one particular defeat that I will never forget, because it came at one of the most important moments of my life: it was the defeat that pushed me forward.

I entered my first fitness competition in June 2013, in Orlando, Florida. While I was training for it, Jimmy kept saying that I needed to do more cardio but I paid no attention to what he said, just because I wanted to antagonize him. But sure enough, once the day of the competition came around and I thought I was in great shape . . . I came in last. Not second or third, but last. I was devastated. In the car on the way back home to Miami I cried the entire time because I felt that I had made huge sacrifices and I had expected to finish in a better position.

Suddenly Jimmy—maybe because he was tired of my attitude—said something I'll never forget. He said: "This type of competition isn't for you. You weren't born for this. You'd better find something else to do, because you clearly can't do this and you have no future here." And at that exact moment, outraged and with tears streaming down my face, I felt as though a giant dragon, one of those that spit fire, finally awoke inside me. I said to Jimmy: "I'm going to show you how I become number one, the best, and I never ever want you to say that again for the rest of your life." That moment marked the beginning of my most radical transformation. I started eating right and I began to train like a beast. From then on, over the following two years, I attended fitness competitions every month and always ended in first or second place.

My first defeat was the beginning of my path to success. I transformed my pain into rage and my rage into the strength to do cardio and weight training while maintaining an ironclad discipline when it came to eating.

One month after that first defeat, in July 2013, I participated in the NPC Southern States 2013 Bikini Novice/Class B competition and came in second among more than one hundred women registered in the same category. In just one month, I was able to change my entire body. I was focused like never before: I ate right, did my cardio, and became obsessed with proving to myself and to Jimmy that I was going to fulfill my promise, and absolutely everyone was impressed with the change. Including me!

Then, during the following four weeks, I continued to train and in August 2013 I participated in the Tampa Bay Pro Show competition, one of the most competitive and demanding events in the North American fitness world. I won the overall competition, which means I got first place in all categories, among all competitors. And from then on, I competed once a month for two years, reaching heights I had never even dreamed of.

## I NO LONGER COMPETE. NOW I JUST WANT TO MOTIVATE YOU. . . .

I spent two years participating in competitions every month. I ultimately stopped competing because it's not healthy to maintain such a low body-fat percentage for so long. Competing professionally is also very stressful, which meant I wasn't happy. You have to follow an extreme diet plan, restricting your water and salt intake, which meant I had to stay away from any social situation so as not to fall into temptation . . . and that was definitely not healthy for my body or my mind. I competed for two years with the sole purpose of proving to myself and to Jimmy that I was capable of getting first place.

But I think that my biggest reward during that time was finding out that when I want something with all my heart, I am capable of achieving it. I stopped competing, but I still train and take care of my body in order to continue my career as a fitness model. And that brings us to today. Today I want to motivate you, along with all my social media followers around the world, to change your lives.

## FITNESS IS MY LIFE

I'm constantly sharing my workout plans through social media, and now, in this book, you will finally have access to my meal plans. My aspiration is to motivate and help women to achieve a strong, toned, feminine body, without going overboard and becoming bulky like a man. I want them to become their best selves. I don't want anyone to aspire to be like me—quite the opposite: I want every woman to dream of being herself, just shining at her absolute brightest.

I was able to become the best version of myself because I was constant, disciplined, and focused. This is so important. You have to work, work, work every day. There's no giving up, no excuses, no veering off the path you have set out for yourself. I don't strive to imitate anyone, and neither should you. I am who I am, I don't pretend to be anyone else, and I don't wear masks. What you see on social media is what you get when you meet me in person.

Health is strength and harmony—looking good and feeling like your body can do whatever you ask of it are priceless. If you want to change your body, you have to start by making the decision, finding your true motives, and working at it like you never have before.

How strong is your passion?

Why are you here?

What's really motivating you to change your body?

Now these are the questions you need to ask yourself. Think hard about your answers before moving on to the next chapter, because once you're in the thick of it, you won't be able to go back to your old habits. Very soon, your old self will begin to disappear.

But that's what you wanted, right?

# 2.

# BEAT THE ENEMY: YOUR MIND AND YOUR BAD HABITS

Do you want to know who your biggest enemy is?
Look in the mirror. Defeat him and the others will flee.

—MIKHAIL LITVAK

**I decided to open** this section of the book with Mikhail Litvak's powerful words because without motivation, your dreams will remain dreams for the rest of your life. Motivation is the engine that will push you, day after day, to get out of bed in order to train, eat right, and control all those self-sabotaging impulses that will try to throw you off course.

I want you to realize that right now you aren't the way you want to be precisely because of the silly excuses you make up for yourself. Yes, I said *excuses*, because when something is a priority for you, you find the space and the time to do it, even if that means getting up at the break of dawn. It all comes down to priorities.

We all have the same twenty-four hours in a day. The only difference is in how we spend our time. If your body and your health are not your priority, then there will never be time to work out and plan your meals. I promised you an

> You can transform your body forever—everyone can. All you need to know is just how much you are willing to give.
>
> —MICHELLE LEWIN

honest book, because honesty is what I'm about. And that's why I have to tell you that the first thing you need to think about is just how much en-

> **You don't have to look like me; all you have to look like is a better version of yourself.**
>
> **—MICHELLE LEWIN**

ergy and time you are willing to put into this plan, because that's what will determine your results.

I won't lie to you and say that if you walk thirty minutes a day, you will achieve a toned and fit body. The path to burning fat and achieving muscle definition is determined 70 percent by what you eat, 20 percent by how you exercise, and 10 percent by how you supplement. If one of the elements in this formula fails, you aren't going to achieve the results you expect. It's that simple.

So think about it—how much are you really willing to put in? Because if you aren't willing to invest the time, passion, and effort I'm going to ask of you, then don't expect to get a six-pack or beautifully toned legs. All I want is for you to clearly understand that the magnitude of your achievements will depend on how much time and energy you invest.

Before we go any further, I want you to do me a very special favor: turn off your inner critic. Forget all the nonsense you say to yourself and ignore anyone who has criticized or made fun of you. Forget the ridiculous advice you get from others that has made you hate yourself. Stop hating and rejecting yourself. You are wonderful and so is your body: you are not and you will never be perfect. No one is. Believe it or not, there are still several aspects of my body that I don't like and would like to improve.

Don't obsess over achieving a perfect body. Instead live to enjoy a harmonious, strong, and above all healthy body. Love yourself and treat your body like a piece of marble from which you will carve a beautiful sculpture. That's why I keep talking about becoming your best self, made entirely by you. You're already beautiful; all you need is to get rid of the excess fat, guilt, and sadness of the past.

> **If you don't love yourself enough, start now and your journey will be easier.**
>
> **—MICHELLE LEWIN**

## FIND A REASON

You can transform your body forever—everyone can. All you need to know is just how much you're willing to give. And more importantly why you want to do it. It's important that you be honest with yourself and look for a real motive, something big and strong—something worthy of you. If you don't have a good reason, something exciting that will really add value to your life, you're going to end up abandoning the fight. That's why I'm asking you to think hard, dream big, and see yourself as your best self: radiant, beautiful, strong. I always say, it's free to dream! And you need to dream before you can make your dreams come true.

If you don't have a strong motive, you won't be strong. It's that simple. Your strength comes from your heart and from a focused mind, not from your current fitness level or the shape of your body. Motivation is the fuel we need in order to join the gym for the first time, which, by the way, is the most difficult step. If you're doing it because you want to wear a dress, look good for a few days in a bathing suit, or go out on a date with that guy you like, those are short-lived reasons. They can inspire you for a while, but the truth is, you're going to have to reevaluate them or change them if you want to go further.

It's easy for me to stay motivated, because being a fitness model is my job; it's the way I make a living. The gym is my office and I simply have to show up at least twice a day. But if this isn't your situation, here's a trick that may help you stay motivated: make a list of the reasons why you want to transform your body.

Think about them, write them down, imagine that you have reached your goal, and visualize how you want to look every day when you get up in the morning. Visualize your new life until it feels so good in your mind that you feel like you have already accomplished it. The mind is very powerful, so you must fill it with good ideas and exciting and positive motives.

**When you feel like giving up, think about why you started.**

**—MICHELLE LEWIN**

Make a list and put it somewhere you will see it every day. If you want you can use images—choose figures that inspire you to continue working toward your goals. Again, remember, this isn't something you can do just because you want to please someone, get a certain guy's attention, or look good for a beach holiday. If your motives are insufficient, your efforts will be too. Try to make your motivation bulletproof. Make it strong and beautiful like you.

One of the most important reasons why I wanted to succeed in life was to be reunited with my family: I wanted my siblings to be able to come to the United States so we could work together toward our common goal. It was the love of my family that led me to a career in fitness. I wanted to become a legal resident in this country, and since becoming a recognized athlete would allow me to achieve that dream, that's what I was going to do. I wanted my family to be together again.

> **Your list of reasons will always keep you on track, or help you refocus whenever you let yourself down.**
>
> **—MICHELLE LEWIN**

Another one of my great reasons has been my love for Jimmy. I want to make him proud of and happy with the enormous amount of work he has put into motivating me, asking me not to eat that piece of pizza because it would throw me off track, demanding that I train my upper body or do more cardio. Jimmy inspired me to change my life, and he introduced me to two beautiful worlds: the world of travel and the world of fitness. This fun Swedish guy is one of the most powerful motivating forces in my life.

Now it's your turn. Write each and every one of the reasons you have to transform your body, from the most trivial to the most heartfelt. Write them here.

My reasons for transforming my body are:

_____

_____

_____

_____

_____

_____

_____

Remember to always keep your list of reasons within reach. It will help you remain focused, and you can turn to it every time you feel listless, depressed, or unmotivated.

# EVERY WEEK COUNTS

As you will see later when you start the meal plan, each week is dedicated to a specific energy, and I have created motivational messages for each day of the plan.

- **Week 1:** Jump-Start with Joy
  Anytime we start a new diet, we embark on it with lots of motivation and a good attitude. We want to change everything we don't like at once, so it's hard to lose motivation in the first week. At this point, the gas tank is full.

- **Week 2:** Motivation and Energy
  By the time the second week rolls around, we start feeling lighter and happier because we were able to make it past the first week. We're still motivated and happy—we are proud of our efforts. We've used up a good part of the gas, but the tank is still mostly full!

- **Week 3:** Discipline and Consistency
  By the third week, challenges start to arise because our bodies will beg us to return to the foods we were accustomed to. At this point we must remain disciplined and consistent in order to stay on track. This new way of eating is not as exciting as it was at first, but we know we need to power through. Here the gas is beginning to run out, and you're going to need to add some more. But once you get through your first twenty-one continuous days, you'll be very likely to achieve great results.

- **Week 4:** Celebration and Reward
  If you were able to get through the first three weeks, by the fourth you will have no trouble getting through your everyday plan and you will celebrate your strength and focus. You will celebrate every day that you have managed to stay on track and the results will speak for themselves. You will feel invincible. You will realize that you've succeeded, and if you have not yet reached your final goal, you can restart the twenty-eight-day cycle as many times as necessary in order to get to where you want to be.

## DON'T GO THROUGH IT ALONE

True, the journey is a lot easier when your partner or your family supports you. If you happen to be married to a man who loves pasta and sweets and keeps the fridge and pantry fully stocked, or if he likes to eat several days a week at fast-food restaurants and asks you to accompany him . . . yes, I can see how that would make weight loss more difficult, but even so, you can't let it defeat you. Try to get your partner to support you or get a group of friends or family together who share your goal, to help you stay focused.

> I achieve anything I want with focus, work, passion, discipline, and perseverance.
>
> —MICHELLE LEWIN

Every day when I go out on the street I have to fight the temptation to eat sweets (in my house there are none!), especially cheesecake, which I love. Like you, I have days when I don't want to get up in the morning to exercise. It happens to all of us. But I have overcome my barriers because I have valuable reasons. I'm disciplined and I'm a perfectionist and I have two defects that have become my best friends: I am both proud and stubborn. I've put these two little devils to work for me—they help me tackle the long and challenging road to fitness with strength, pride, and passion because I don't want to be defeated. My body will do what I want it to do, not the other way around.

> DON'T GIVE UP! If you fall, quickly get back up and get back on track. It's the only way to get there!
>
> —MICHELLE LEWIN

## TELL ME THERE'S SOMETHING I CAN'T DO, AND THEN SIT DOWN AND WATCH ME DO IT

I have the strength not to be defeated. I am persistent, fierce, and competitive. Perhaps that is one of my great secrets: I decide what battles I want to fight, I hold on to my powerful motives, and I throw myself into the hard work without ever thinking of giving up. I never do.

My dreams come true because I plan for them. I am a normal person; sometimes I get up in the morning and I don't want to go to the gym, but then I feel that if I don't

**When you think you can't give it any more, keep going. That's what sets you apart from everyone else.**

**—MICHELLE LEWIN**

go, it is one less day on my path to achieving my goals and objectives. The hardest part is the first step—just leaving the house. But once you get out and jump on the treadmill, you've gotten past the hardest part. That's why I will always say that you must have a strong mind in order to have a strong body. Being fit starts with your vision and your passion, and only once you have a positive and committed mind-set does this journey become sweat, strength, and muscle.

## DITCH THE DRAMA

I want to continue to inspire you to believe that anything is possible, that you can change your mind and your body, overcome your weaknesses, and become your best self. Because anything is possible as long as it's what you want and you decide to do.

**You can achieve anything, as long as you really want it.**

**—MICHELLE LEWIN**

Don't complain; don't cry; don't let anyone give you silly consolations when you're being weak. If Jimmy had consoled me after I lost that first competition, today I would be a loser. His hard words burned me; they made me a warrior whose pride was hurt. That pain turned into sweat, then into successes, travels, and much happiness.

If you've missed opportunities, stop wallowing in what has already happened and remember that there will always be new ones; you just need to keep your eyes open and your body ready to act and become

**When you want something, declare it, work for it, and you will see it come true.**

**—MICHELLE LEWIN**

strong. That's what fitness is about. And you're the one who decides when to start.

## TREAT YOUR BODY LIKE A TEMPLE, NOT A GARBAGE DUMP

Your body needs to be the right support for your mind and spirit. If you care for it, your body can take you where you want to go with all the power you need to get there.

Remember, you must have powerful motives, a well-focused mind that can ignore negative comments, and above all, a body that receives the best food and rest possible.

Give your body "the best fuel," so that it can become a fat-burning, muscle-making machine. Always take your body to the limit but don't forget to allow it to rest and give yourself the opportunity to relax, laugh, and spend time with others. Life isn't just about competing; it's about love and sharing your passion. The competition is never against others; it's always against yourself. It's about striving to become your best self—drawing strength to overcome pain, fear, and laziness; pushing yourself to the limit of your mental and physical capacity so that you can shine like a diamond.

## TWO MORE TIPS BEFORE YOU GET STARTED

1. You need to give yourself realistic goals. You need to take it one day at a time. Stay focused and motivated and don't expect fast results. When you're pulling the weeds off the side of the road on your way to your final goal, you shouldn't keep your eyes on your target but on the weeds you are pulling—that's how you'll do well and minimize the risks.

2. Don't let gossips, haters, or losers turn your mind into a garbage dump. You'll always encounter people who don't believe in you. Don't let anyone rob you of your dreams or flood your mind with negative thoughts, criticism, or mockery. Never let anyone tell you that there's something you can't do. You're the only one who knows how far you want to go. But you always have to fight for what you want.

Are you ready? Are you motivated?

Move on to the next chapter to learn the five most important things to know before you change your lifestyle.

Let the party begin!

# 3.

# FIVE THINGS YOU NEED TO KNOW BEFORE YOU CHANGE YOUR LIFESTYLE

**W**e've all dreamed of having that slim, toned body we see in magazines. But have you ever wondered how much time and effort it took that girl in the magazine to look the way she does? I'm sure you haven't. Seeing the results and admiring them is easy. But it takes patience, discipline, and courage to achieve them.

If you are thinking of adopting fitness as a lifestyle and not just as a trend, then this chapter is for you. This is where I'll tell you everything you need to know as well as what you should and shouldn't do.

To become your best self, look good, and feel fabulous, here are five things you need to know:

## 1. FITNESS IS NO CHILD'S PLAY

Although many believe that fitness athletes are attracted to this discipline out of vanity, they aren't aware of the huge sacrifice the lifestyle entails. So I'm going to tell you. I want you to know every detail and be sure of every step you take. First, I'll tell you a little about this world, which is now my world: the world of fitness.

Back in the day, the word *fitness* was used to refer to the physical activities—performed at a gym—that exercised the entire body and worked all the muscle groups in order to achieve good body composition, strength, flexibility, and endurance. Later, the term began to be used to indicate a general state of health and well-being that could be achieved by leading a healthy lifestyle, mainly through exercise. Either way, the goal of fitness has always been to promote a person's well-being, which is ultimately what we all want!

Fitness can bring you many benefits, the most important of which is being able to maintain a strong and healthy body and mind.

## WHAT CHANGES CAN YOU EXPECT?

1. You will achieve a balance in your body structure by maintaining your proportion of muscles, fat, bones, and organs in perfect harmony.
2. You will improve your aerobic endurance: thanks to this, your heart and your entire cardiovascular system will work more efficiently. This is your machine's engine.
3. You will increase your resistance and muscular strength, affecting everything from how you carry grocery bags to how you hold your children or your pets.
4. You will increase your flexibility. This will allow you to keep your joints healthy and move freely.
5. You will improve your self-esteem. Feeling good is more important than looking good, but looking good will certainly help you feel comfortable and enjoy your body freely and without fear.

## WHAT DO YOU NEED TO GET STARTED?

Desire, patience, and discipline! It's about changing your lifestyle—a change you probably won't accomplish in just a couple of days. You will have to devote time and effort to changing what you have been doing for years into something completely different. Fitness requires dedication, preparation, and above all, motivation.

## ARE THERE ANY RISKS?

Not everyone is in optimal health; therefore, you should certainly take some precautionary measures before you radically change what you have been doing up until now. If you are unhealthy, suffer from an illness (such as obesity, diabetes, high blood pressure, stroke, high cholesterol, or elevated triglycerides), from limitations in your bones or joints; if you have unhealthy habits such as drinking or smoking; if you are sedentary or have never exercised before, you should seek medical advice before starting any plan.

## IS THERE A DIFFERENCE BETWEEN BEING FIT AND BEING HEALTHY?

Definitely not! *Fitness* means well-being. Being fit is synonymous with being healthy—both inside and out.

## DO I NEED TO ENTER COMPETITIONS IN ORDER TO BE FIT?

No, the truth is that competitions are for those who like them. You can certainly adopt fitness as your lifestyle without having to compete in anything related to fitness or bodybuilding. Besides, they are totally different disciplines.

Traditional bodybuilding aims at increasing muscle mass and having very little body fat. In bodybuilding competitions there is a comparison round in which competitors are asked to take the stage and stand side by side as they perform a series of poses that highlight their muscle definition and balance. There is another round during which contestants have to perform a specific posing routine to music.

On the other hand, in fitness competitions, competitors are looking to achieve a stylized and athletic appearance. They train to reduce their body fat percentage without gaining too much muscle mass. Women compete in two-piece swimsuits with heels. There is a music routine round in which competitors show their strength, flexibility and training program.

## 2. EXCESS FAT IS YOUR MAIN ENEMY

The desire to lose weight, get rid of those extra rolls, and optimize their figure is usually what pushes women to enter the world of fitness. But oftentimes we don't realize that behind the things we want to change are the consequences of what we have been doing wrong for years.

Being overweight is a serious health problem that almost always takes a toll. And in order to correct it, you need to act responsibly and seek out the right help, without resorting to crazy fad diets, extreme exercise routines, magic pills, or miracle injections.

Let's start by taking a look at our body's three main components:

1. Lean mass: the body's muscles, organs, and bones. Men have a greater muscle mass than women.
2. Fat: despite the bad rap, our bodies need a certain amount of fat in order to perform certain functions. Fat is where we store our energy, and it also strengthens and protects our joints, nerves, and organs and performs important hormonal functions, which I will tell you more about later.
3. Water: water is the largest component of total body weight (50 to 60 percent of our body is water) and it's inside and outside our cells.

It's important that you understand that when you get on your scale, you aren't weighing only your fat—you're weighing your entire body. Bones and organs do not vary much in weight, but water, muscles, and fat do.

There is a "traditional" way of measuring obesity—the body mass index (BMI), which is calculated by dividing your weight in kilograms over your height squared in meters (BMI = weight in kilograms/height in meters$^2$). To bring your weight in pounds to kilograms, just divide the pounds by 2.2.

To convert your height in feet/inches to meters, use the following table:

| FEET/INCHES | METERS |
|:---:|:---:|
| 4'0" | 1.22 |
| 4'1" | 1.24 |
| 4'2" | 1.27 |
| 4'3" | 1.30 |

| FEET/INCHES | METERS |
| --- | --- |
| 4'4" | 1.32 |
| 4'5" | 1.35 |
| 4'6" | 1.37 |
| 4'7" | 1.40 |
| 4'8" | 1.42 |
| 4'9" | 1.45 |
| 4'10" | 1.47 |
| 4'11" | 1.50 |
| 5'0" | 1.52 |
| 5'1" | 1.55 |
| 5'2" | 1.57 |
| 5'3" | 1.60 |
| 5'4" | 1.63 |
| 5'5" | 1.65 |
| 5'6" | 1.68 |
| 5'7" | 1.70 |
| 5'8" | 1.73 |
| 5'9" | 1.75 |
| 5'10" | 1.78 |
| 5'11" | 1.80 |
| 6'0" | 1.83 |
| 6'1" | 1.85 |
| 6'2" | 1.88 |
| 6'3" | 1.91 |
| 6'4" | 1.93 |
| 6'5" | 1.96 |
| 6'6" | 1.98 |
| 6'7" | 2.01 |
| 6'8" | 2.03 |
| 6'9" | 2.06 |
| 6'10" | 2.08 |
| 6'11" | 2.11 |

If you only know your weight in pounds, you can use the following formula:

$$BMI = weight\ [in\ pounds]\ /\ height\ [in\ inches]^2\ x\ 703$$

Calculate your BMI by dividing your weight in pounds by your height in inches (squared) and multiply the result by 703.

For example:

Weight = 150 pounds, height = 5′5″ (65″)
$$BMI = [150 \div (65)^2]\ x\ 703 = 24.96$$

Now that you have your BMI, you can use the following table to see how overweight or obese you really are:

| CATEGORY | BODY MASS INDEX (BMI) |
|---|---|
| Underweight | Less than 18.5 |
| Normal Range | 18.5–24.9 |
| Overweight | 25.0–29.9 |
| Obese | Over 30.0 |

However, this measure doesn't work for everyone, and it is especially uninstructive for fitness and bodybuilding athletes who have high BMIs due to the fact that a large percentage of their weight comes from their muscles. A BMI measurement doesn't differentiate fat from muscle mass.

So, what do we do in those cases? Well, there are a few other options to measure your body-fat percentage, such as skinfold testing (also known as caliper testing) and bioelectrical impedance analysis (both can be performed by a nutritionist or health professional). With either of these tests you can get a detailed body-composition report, including your body-fat percentage.

## BODY-FAT PERCENTAGE

In this table you will find the normal body-fat percentage range depending on your age:

| AGE | WOMEN (%) | MEN (%) |
|---|---|---|
| 15–20 | 18–22 | 15–18 |
| 21–25 | 21–23 | 16–20 |
| 26–30 | 22–24 | 19–21 |
| 31–35 | 24–26 | 20–21 |
| 36–45 | 25–27 | 21–23 |
| 46–50 | 28–30 | 22–23 |
| 51–60 | 29–31 | 23–24 |
| >60 | 29–31 | 24–25 |

Now, if you're competing it's a whole different ballpark. Your fat percentage values should be even lower, for better muscle definition. For competitions, athletes strive to be within the following ranges:

| | WOMEN | MEN |
|---|---|---|
| Essential Fat | 10–12% | 2–4% |
| Athletes | 14–20% | 6–13% |
| Fitness | 21–24% | 14–17% |

Our bodies store fat in two different ways:

▶ **Visceral fat** is lodged in the muscles, central nervous system, organs, and bone marrow and covers between 2 percent and 4 percent of total body weight in men, and 10 percent to 12 percent in women because their measurement includes the fat in breast tissues and on hips, where it is necessary for the proper functioning of the reproductive system.

▶ **Subcutaneous fat** is stored as an energy reserve throughout the body. For male athletes, the percentage should be between 6 percent and 13 percent, and in women it should be between 11 percent and 21 percent.

## FORGET YOUR WEIGHT; MEASURE YOUR FAT

Not everyone has access to a nutritionist or health professional who can measure their body-fat percentage. In these cases there's another easy way to find out, and all you need is a tape measure.

You can learn a lot about your body with a simple tape measure. From now on you will record your body measurements on a piece of paper. Be sure to take note of your start date and remember to measure yourself twice a week in order to record your changes. You can quit your obsession with weighing yourself every morning, since your weight can vary depending on several factors, such as your salt intake, whether or not you ate too much or drank too much water, and your hormonal changes. A tape measure, however, will tell you nothing but the truth. If your measurements go down it's because you're losing fat. Period.

### 3. DON'T OVERDO IT

I know I've already said it, but I'll say it again: there is no easy way to do this. I keep saying this because every day I see how people try to cut corners and obtain fast results at a very high risk. As long as you do things right there's no danger in the fitness lifestyle, but you need to take it slowly.

## THE EASIEST SHORTCUT IS THE WORST OF ALL: ANABOLIC STEROIDS

Anabolic steroids are synthetic substances similar to male sex hormones that are used to aid muscle growth (anabolic effects) and the development of male sexual characteristics in both men and women. These substances were created to treat hypogonadism, a disease in which the testicles are unable to produce enough of the male hormone (testosterone) necessary for the normal growth, development, and functioning of the body. But when scientists discovered the effects these steroids had on muscle growth, bodybuilders and other athletes began to use them in an abusive and illicit manner.

The main reasons why people use steroids are to improve their performance, increase muscle mass, and reduce body fat. Some anabolic steroids come in the form of pills, others in the form of injections, and yet others come in the form of ointments (gels) or creams that are rubbed onto the skin. The doses used may be ten to one hundred times higher than those used for medical reasons, which of course means they can have many negative effects, ranging from acne and breast development in men to life-threatening ones like heart attacks and liver cancer. Most of these effects go away as soon as you stop taking them. Others don't. Believe me, they're terrible.

## IF YOU GO TOO FAST, YOU'LL FALL

When you decide to go too fast, another one of the problems you can encounter is injuring yourself as a result of bad practices, improper use of training equipment, or poor physical condition. The most common injuries are sprains, muscle and tendon tears, knee injuries, swollen muscles, Achilles tendon injuries, pain along the shin, bone fractures, and dislocations.

Never try to "push through" the pain of an injury. Stop exercising immediately, because continuing can only make the injury worse. Some injuries should be examined immediately by your doctor, for example: if you have severe pain, swelling, or numbness in any part of your body; if you are unable to hold any weight in the injured area; if a previous injury hurts or becomes swollen; or if any of your joints feels abnormal or unstable.

If you don't have any of these symptoms, you can treat the injury at home safely, by applying ice locally (with a cold pack or ice pack) for twenty minutes, four to eight times a day. Place compresses on the injured area in order to reduce swelling, and elevate the part of your body with the help of a pillow. And most importantly, make sure you rest. Don't exercise the injured part of your body for the following forty-eight hours, and do your best to cut back on everyday activities.

## HOW CAN YOU PREVENT INJURIES?

▶ Forget about being a "weekend warrior." Don't try to do in one or two days the physical activity you should be doing throughout the week.

- Learn to perform your exercises correctly. This will help reduce the risk of injury. If you don't know how to perform the movements, it's best to seek the help of a coach.
- Know your body's limits and gradually increase the level of exercise. Taking it slow but safe is better than going fast and getting injured.
- Do full-body exercises, such as cardio and other exercises that will increase your strength and flexibility.
- Always do a few warm-up exercises before you begin your weight-training routine. And make sure you stretch at the end of your session.
- Wear appropriate clothing, accessories, and equipment. Do not wrap yourself in girdles, thermal clothing, or accessories that will hinder your movements while you exercise.
- Be just as mindful about your food and water intake as you are about your training. If you want your body to do more, you need to give it the right amount and the right quality of fuel.
- Rest. Most injuries occur when we are tired or exhausted.
- Don't get creative. If there's something you don't know, ask. Don't follow your sister's or your neighbor's training routine. What works for one person might hurt another.

## 4. CHECK YOUR HORMONES BEFORE YOU START

Your entire body is controlled by your hormones. They do all the work. They control your mood, your temperament, your energy level, how much fat you burn, your hair quality, how healthy your skin looks, and even how long it takes for your muscles to recover. It's extremely important to make sure your hormones are working properly before you start an exercise program. Especially after age forty!

If your hormonal system isn't working right, you may have trouble seeing results even if you train and eat properly. Dr. Samar Yorde, my coauthor, experienced this herself. Suddenly, everything that had always worked for her when it came to controlling her weight, and what she applied to her patients with very good results, stopped working for her. She went on strenuous diets and endured grueling workouts; however, her weight loss was minimal, and as soon as she veered off track, even if it was for just a little while, she'd put the weight back on. The problem was in her hormones.

One of the most important hormones in your body is testosterone. Yes, just like men, women have—and need—testosterone. Testosterone levels in women start to decrease when they are about twenty-five years of age, and a woman in her forties will probably have about half the testosterone levels of a woman in her twenties.

Something many women don't know is that when their bodies are lacking in testosterone, they can often experience chronic fatigue, a decreased libido, and even lack of happiness. Yes, when you have low testosterone levels, you lose your sense of well-being. So make sure you keep your eye on this hormone. Testosterone regulates many important processes in the body: it maintains the proper amount of muscle mass and bone density, and it regulates your sleep cycle and your red blood cell count, among other things. As you get older, your testosterone levels drop naturally, but this process can accelerate due to high levels of stress, a poor diet, low levels of vitamin D, weight gain, or a sedentary lifestyle.

## SYMPTOMS OF LOW TESTOSTERONE LEVELS

▶ Decreased vitality
▶ Mood swings
▶ Always feeling tired
▶ Decreased libido
▶ Hot flashes
▶ Bone loss
▶ Loss of muscle mass and strength
▶ Weight gain
▶ Memory loss
▶ Difficulty sleeping

Another hormone you have probably heard about is the human growth hormone (HGH). A drop in this hormone often goes unnoticed. But did you know that HGH is a natural testosterone booster?

If you are feeling depressed, with decreased strength and muscle mass; if you have hair loss or dry skin; if you have difficulty concentrating or you notice that your memory is failing; if you have gained weight, especially around the waist, and you have a decreased sexual desire . . . you need to go to your doctor to get your hormones checked! If your tests come back showing low hormone levels, hormone replacement therapy may be necessary to improve your well-being.

But the good news is that in addition, you can naturally increase these two hormones—testosterone and HGH—if you follow these six steps:

## 1. Exercise with weight training and intervals

If you want to naturally increase your testosterone and HGH levels, you can combine weight training with high-intensity interval training (HIIT). Focusing on weight lifting exercises (eight to twelve repetitions) that involve large muscles—such as quadriceps, femoral, hamstring, back, shoulder, and chest muscles—will help your body to increase these values.

Additionally, interval cardiovascular training is the most effective way to burn the sugar stored in your body (glycogen). It causes your body to burn fat during the following thirty-six hours in order to replace its reserves. In addition to increasing your hormone levels, HIIT can help you burn three to nine times more fat, lower your resting heart rate, lower your blood pressure, keep your brain young by increasing circulation, and stimulate your body's lymphatic system.

## 2. Eat good fats!

Eating excessive amounts of junk food and carbs won't help you improve your hormones. On the other hand, coconut oil; fermented dairy products such as kefir; omega-3 fatty acids; flaxseeds; chia seeds; and avocado, olive, almond, and walnut oils are great allies if you want to increase your testosterone and human growth hormone.

## 3. Watch your vitamin D!

Vitamin $D_3$ is one of the most important nutrients when it comes to increasing your testosterone levels. It's very important to sit in the sun for at least thirty minutes in order to get your daily fix of this vitamin.

## 4. Eliminate sugar!

Excess processed foods and sugar raise your blood glucose levels. This means that in order to maintain normal blood sugar levels, your pancreas has to work overtime to produce insulin, which helps transport blood sugar to your cells, where it can be metabolized. If your cells are bombarded with insulin over an extended period of time, you will develop insulin resistance, which causes type 2 diabetes. And once you develop diabetes, your body is no longer able to produce the levels of testosterone it should be producing.

## 5. Rest well!

Sleep is essential to the proper functioning of our physical and mental capacities. But it's not enough just to sleep. You need to sleep well. The better you sleep, the better you will be able to perform your daily activities. Scientific evidence has shown that a lack of sleep can reduce testosterone and HGH levels.

In addition to sleeping more hours, it's important to be able to sleep soundly. Most of the testosterone and HGH we produce is secreted during the deepest sleep phase (the REM, or rapid eye movement, phase), which is also when the brain is able to recover and rest.

If we don't get enough deep sleep, our bodies end up producing more cortisol—also known as the stress hormone—which will immediately bring changes to our metabolic activity.

## 6. Supplement properly!

Vitamin C, L-arginine, and L-glutamine (I'll tell you about these later) seem to improve HGH values, as well as help you with your performance.

If you are over forty, you absolutely must ask your doctor to check on your hormones. Your hormones might be preventing you from losing weight without your knowing it. Hormones need to be taken very seriously. They cause many unwanted symptoms, as well as hinder and slow down the entire process. Your body needs to be in perfect balance in order for you to reach your desired results.

## 5. IT'S A MARATHON, NOT A SPRINT

This is fitness. It's a lifelong race—a competition between who you were and who you want to be. But above all, it's a competition between the part of you that wants to give up and the part of you that knows you can achieve more.

When you get up every morning wanting to be better, when you spend more time training and taking care of your body, you know you're in the right place. You made the right decision: you've decided to change what you had (body and mind) for what you want. There is no better feeling than looking in the mirror and saying, "I am better than yesterday; I look better than before; I have achieved more than ever."

A building needs a good foundation. And it needs a lot of planning. Like a good engineer, you need to sit down and make the decision to build it. With pencil and paper in hand, design the body you want. Draw the body of your dreams, but try to remain realistic. Don't compare yourself; don't draw someone else. Remember that this is you, but just a better version. Now flip the piece of paper over and write down the five things you need to start doing and five things you need to stop doing in order to achieve this body. Are you done? Then take the piece of paper and START DOING WHAT YOU NEED TO DO. What you are doing wrong will start to change as long as you do what's right.

Just like everyone else, I had a hard time getting started. It took time to understand what I was doing wrong and that I wasn't going to get any results if I wasn't willing to change what I was doing. Your body and your mind will adapt to the changes, but you CAN'T GIVE UP. In a couple of months you'll be grateful that you didn't give up that day, the next, or the following. And when you least expect it, your building will be standing tall.

# 4.

# METABOLISM AND
# ENERGY BALANCE

*Metabolism* **is a** word that gets thrown around a lot. Anyone who has ever been on a diet, either to gain or to lose weight, is familiar with the term. People talk about having a slow metabolism, a fast metabolism, a metabolism that's slowing down, a metabolic disorder . . . For many women it's a real headache to make sense of what it all means. As a fitness athlete I've had to learn all about it, so I'll do my best to explain how it works.

The first thing you need to know is that your metabolism is your internal computer. It's the process by which your body converts food into energy. Your metabolism literally transforms what you eat into the energy your body needs to perform the functions it needs to perform in order to keep you alive. Because even if you're lying in bed doing nothing, your body needs energy to breathe, think, digest food, keep your blood ciculating, and so on.

Internally, your metabolism consists of a series of chemical reactions, some of which are very complex, just like a computer's internal circuits. Even though we can't see them, we know they're there and that they're indispensable to the proper functioning of your body.

Now, the metabolism that your body is always running is called your basal metabolism; it's active even when you are at rest, and its proper functioning depends on your body's muscle mass. Your basal metabolic rate can increase only if you increase your muscle mass, and at the same time, if you lose muscle mass, your basal metabolic rate will decrease. So as we age or when we lose muscle mass due to illness, our metabolism slows down.

The good news is that even though our bodies slow down and burn fewer calories as we lose muscle mass, we have two other ways of burning calories. The first one is by eating. Yes, you read that right. Every time you eat, you burn calories. This is called the thermic effect of food (TEF) and it results from the energy that your body invests in digesting and absorbing what you eat. When you eat carbohydrates or fats this effect increases by 5 percent, but when you eat proteins the rate at which you burn calories increases by up to 25 percent. We'll talk more about this later.

Last but not least, we burn calories while exercising. If we add up your basal metabolic rate, your TEF, and the effect of exercise . . . that's a whole lot of calories burned during the day.

For reasons still unknown, each body seems to have a "magic weight," a number that the body always seeks to maintain. If you try to deviate from that weight your body struggles to come back to that magic number. For example, when you are trying to lose weight and you restrict the calories you eat, your magic weight comes into play and your body lowers your basal metabolic rate by lowering the number of calories you burn over the course of twenty-four hours, as if it wants to protect you from a state of deprivation.

In order to defend yourself from your body's self-sabotaging efforts, you must compensate for the situation. How? Reduce the calories you are eating, and go out and burn more calories through exercise. This is the key.

## IS IT POSSIBLE TO CHANGE MY COMPUTER?

Your metabolism is determined by several factors, such as your genetics, your body composition (percentage of muscle mass and fat), your gender, your hormonal health, your activity level, and your age. Some of these factors are within your control and you can modify them (your muscle mass and activity level, for example), while others you can do nothing about (such as your genetics and your age).

How can you find out whether your metabolism is working at full speed? There are certain signs that may point to a slow metabolism, such as chronic fatigue, feeling cold all the time, hair loss, dry skin, brittle nails, difficulty sleeping through the night, difficulty concentrating, constipation, feeling bloated after eating, anxiety, having difficulty losing weight, and frequent infections, among others.

## WHY DOES ONE'S METABOLISM SLOW DOWN?

You'll be surprised to hear that you're probably the one to blame for this. Yes, one of the main causes of a slow metabolism is a bad diet.

In order to stay balanced, our bodies need to eat constantly and get enough rest. At the cellular level, your metabolism's pathways depend on the nutrients you offer them. You need to get a variety of nutrients, including proteins, carbohydrates, fats, fatty acids, and vitamins, to produce the energy that is then used by the body to build, maintain, and repair itself.

Very low-calorie diets don't give your body its key nutrients; they rob the body of the raw materials it needs. The factory stops. This is why these diets start well but end badly. At first you lose weight at an alarming speed, but then you get stuck when your body detects that it's starving and calorie deprived. Your body can't differentiate between "on purpose" hunger, and disease and illness hunger. The result? Out of fear that you may once again deprive it of food, it clings to every calorie you eat. Whether you eat a piece of lettuce or a french fry, everything is stored as energy—as FAT.

And not only do you get fat; you get sick too. The lack of calories from a strict and unbalanced diet translates into less fuel for your body's systems, and it's just a question of time before they stop working. Low-calorie diets tend to lead to frequent colds, problems with your reproductive system, mood swings, and infections.

## STOP EXTREME DIETING!

Give your body the calories it needs. Don't deprive your body of what it needs, because hormonal and cellular changes actually activate your hunger and thirst instincts and reduce your ability to burn fat and grow muscle. Give your body the high-quality calories it needs; don't feed it junk.

When you eat right you have better digestion, you feel good, and you are able to stay motivated. Eating enough is essential to feeling active and to being able to gain strength and muscle mass faster. You will also feel less tired and more willing to work out.

Eating right will help you embark on this journey in peace and without agonizing over everything you put in your mouth. Depriving yourself of everything can increase your anxiety and your cravings for "forbidden" foods. One of the best ways to keep your metabolism active throughout the day is to eat. You shouldn't skip meals such as breakfast or dinner in order to reduce your caloric intake—this is a terrible idea, since your systems will immediately stop working.

## REST UP!

Another terrible mistake is to believe that spending hours upon hours at the gym will accelerate your metabolism. Nothing could be further from the truth. When your body feels the excess, the fatigue, and the lack of rest, it begins to shut down, just like when you put your computer in "sleep mode." It's a way of conserving energy. Make sure you exercise enough, but don't exercise too much. A good training session that lasts one to two hours, at most, is ideal. Also, remember how important it is to rest and sleep to keep your hormones—testosterone, growth hormone, and cortisol—under control so as not to allow your body to store more fat. In addition to gaining weight you can cause your body to resist insulin, which will in turn disrupt your blood sugar levels.

## EXERCISE EFFICIENTLY!

Train smart. You can achieve a much higher performance and metabolic impact if you add HIIT to your routine. Adding intervals that go from a greater effort—such as increasing the speed on the treadmill—and then slowing it down activates your metabolism better than if you just get on the treadmill for a brisk walk. HIIT has a prolonged effect on your metabolism because it helps the body to continue burning calories long after you've finished your workout.

One of the best things about HIIT is that it requires less time than traditional cardio. And, as if that weren't enough, you burn more fat. Your body needs higher levels of oxygen to recover after intense activity. These workouts are also effective in improving your cardiovascular function, and they help with insulin sensitivity, decrease cortisol levels, and improve respiratory resistance and muscle endurance.

## NO ACTIVE METABOLISM WITHOUT WEIGHTS!

As I told you, your basal metabolic rate depends on how much muscle mass you have, so if you don't strengthen your muscles, your basal metabolic rate will plummet. To gain muscle you have to weight train without fear—and you have to do it consistently, not just from time to time. If you aren't constantly stimulating your muscles, there will be no growth. If you're trying to gain muscle fast, I recommend lifting heavy weights for eight to twelve repetitions, for forty-five minutes five days a week. There's no result without effort. There's no metabolism without strength training.

## STOP EATING JUNK FOOD!

Filling your body with inflammatory, sugary, fatty, processed foods is the equivalent of loading your computer with viruses. And in the same way your computer would start to slow down, your body will too. By eating junk food you cause terrible damage to your body and accelerate the aging of your cells. Your body recognizes processed and inflammatory foods as toxins, so when you eat them you trigger your immune system's fight-or-flight response, which in turn increases the production of stress hormones, and your metabolism slows down. Even some foods that are labeled as "healthy" are to blame for weight gain, fatigue, hormone imbalance, and digestive problems.

Stay away from sugary drinks (including soft drinks and juices), processed foods made from grains—especially those containing gluten (including wheat products such as bread, pasta, cereals, crackers, muffins, desserts, chips, and granola bars)—refined vegetable oils, artificial sweeteners, low-quality dairy products, and high-fat animal products.

*Juices and drinks:* When you put fruit in the blender, you completely destroy the fiber it contains and turn it into a glass full of sugar. Not to mention that the sugary, processed commercial versions come packed with calories. You should also stay away from other sources of hidden sugars, such as alcoholic beverages, bottled caffeinated drinks, energy drinks, cereals, whole dairy products, and bottled dressings. Sugar is everywhere, hidden under names like corn syrup, dextrose, fructose, juice concentrate, maltodextrin, raw sugar, brown sugar, and so on.

*Refined grains and bread:* When consumed in excess, refined grains can cause inflammation and damage to your digestive system, primarily because of the amount of starch and gluten they contain. For women who aren't very active and are prone to gaining weight, starch can quickly turn into sugar and cause cravings. Whole grain products also contain gluten, as well as added sugar, salt, and synthetic preservatives, and they are oftentimes "fortified" with synthetic vitamins and minerals that can be difficult to metabolize, having the same effects as refined products.

*Oils and fats:* Selecting the wrong kind and amount of fat may end up interfering with your ability to regulate your appetite, your mood, your hormone production, and your digestion. Simply put, all your efforts can go to waste. Most commercially sold vegetable oils are combined with solvents such as hexane during the manufacturing process, and it's still unclear whether there are any health risks associated with the use of these solvents. When used in processed foods these oils can also cause inflammation throughout the body, disrupting metabolism. The best oils will always be olive oil, avocado oil, and coconut oil.

*"Light" products:* So-called "healthy" and "light" snacks are usually bombs prepared with processed vegetable oils (including safflower or sunflower oils), refined carbohydrates, and sodium. And depending on the kind, these ultraprocessed foods can also contain trans fats, such as partially hydrogenated oils, which can cause many health problems, such as inflammation, and slow down your metabolism.

*Artificial sweeteners, the worst offenders:* Of all the terrible foods, this one takes the prize. Artificial sweeteners, including aspartame and sucralose, are probably the most misleading of all. They boast "no calories" and "no guilt," which makes them sound appealing, but these artificial substances alter your antioxidant system, age your body, and oxidize it. They also stimulate your appetite and increase carbohydrate cravings. Their manufacturers claim they save you calories but that ends up being a lie, since they increase your appetite and actually cause you to eat more.

Switch to stevia, the only natural zero-calorie sweetener—it's a product of the stevia plant, and it's three hundred times sweeter than sugar.

## GIVE YOUR BODY THE BEST!

I know you've read a lot about foods that are claimed to be "metabolism boosters." I hate to be the one to disappoint you, but metabolism boosters don't exist. They're nothing but an excuse for losers, the "solution" they turn to when they simply don't want to exercise. Remember, there is no easy fix, and if you don't exercise you won't see any changes to your metabolism. No matter how many spices you eat, how much green tea or caffeine you drink, you simply won't see results unless you exercise. In fact, you'll end up with terrible digestive problems.

Now, that isn't to say that certain foods can't help your body use its energy better. The thermic effect of some foods varies, and your body works harder to break down and metabolize certain foods (such as proteins!). Other foods can help you because of their anti-inflammatory properties and because they can help slow your cells' aging process. When your cells remain young and efficient, your metabolism will stay active longer.

## GOOD PROTEINS

It's extremely important to eat proteins. It takes your body a little longer to digest proteins than processed foods, and you will burn a few more calories while your digestive system is at work. But keep in mind that they need to be high-quality, low-fat proteins. Because, believe me, a piece of fried chicken will definitely have many more calories than what your body can burn! There is zero benefit to you.

But beyond the fact that doing so can help you burn more calories, eating protein helps you delay hunger and stay satiated, which will help you have better control over the portions you eat. You won't be so hungry by the time you reach your next meal and you will be able to prepare your food with intelligence, not despair. Besides, proteins keep you energized and help stabilize blood sugar while also helping build the muscle mass that's actually responsible for burning the calories.

## GREEN TEA

Green tea has so many benefits: it's loaded with antioxidants and is proven to have thermogenic properties that promote weight loss. The benefits of green tea are: reducing fat absorption, stimulating satiety, and increasing thermogenesis, which translates into weight loss. Drinking two to four cups a day may help the body burn 17 percent more calories.

## SPICES

Foods that naturally "warm up" your body, such as cayenne pepper, chili, and other spices, contain an active compound called capsaicin that raises your body temperature while slightly stimulating your metabolism. Other spices such as cinnamon, pepper, and ginger help burn fat and decrease your appetite, so they can help you lose weight too.

Finally, I want to tell you about apple cider vinegar, one of my favorite ingredients for salads. Apple cider vinegar stimulates your metabolism, prevents aging, improves digestion, balances blood sugars, and boosts your metabolism by helping your body use nutrients better.

This is one of my favorite chapters! If you apply these tips to a T, without any doubt and without fear of being wrong, you will turn your body into a great fat-burning machine. Use everything you've learned! And now let's dive into the topic of food, which, as I mentioned before, constitutes 70 percent of what it takes to achieve the body of your dreams.

# HOW TO REV UP YOUR METABOLISM

| WHAT SLOWS DOWN YOUR METABOLISM | HOW TO REV IT BACK UP AGAIN |
|---|---|
| Aging: You lose muscle mass as you age. You will lose about 2 to 3% of your metabolism per decade of life. | Exercise every day: Train with weights and do your cardio in order to maintain your muscle mass and keep your metabolism going. |
| Lack of sleep: Your metabolism slows down in order to preserve energy. | Sleep more! at least 7 hours a day. |
| Lack of strength training: Doing cardio will help you keep your body-fat percentage under control but it won't help you gain muscle mass, and the less muscle mass you have, the lower your metabolism. | Pump some iron: Lift weights at least 3 times a week. Don't be afraid to add weight in order to do fewer repetitions, otherwise your muscles won't grow. |
| Cardio only: When you do cardio, your body remains active during the 2 following hours, burning more and more calories. | Weights and cardio: If you do both cardio and weight training you will have a super-active metabolism for much longer. When you lift weights your body remains active and burning calories for 48 to 72 more hours. |
| Traditional cardio: Moderate exercise will help you maintain your current weight, but it's not so effective when it comes to burning calories and fat. | High-intensity interval training (HIIT): HIIT will give your metabolism a boost during and after your training session. Besides, it's great if you don't have much time to exercise. If you ramp up the intensity you can cut back on time. |
| Diet saboteurs: Fruit juice, carbs, artificial sweeteners, and fried and processed foods. They all contain toxins that will slow down and unbalance your hormones, causing inflammation. | Stimulants: Natural, fresh, whole foods; high-quality proteins, legumes, fruits, vegetables, and stevia (instead of sugar). |

# 5.

# FOODS THAT CAN TRANSFORM YOUR BODY

**W**e've talked about your metabolism, how your body works, and how that wonderful machine is capable of transforming every mouthful of food into pure energy. Now, it's not enough to have a machine that works. For it to work efficiently, you need to provide it with quality raw materials in the right amounts.

It's important that you not only eat, but nurture and build yourself from within. For that to happen you need to select the right foods and ensure that you receive the macronutrients (proteins, fats, and carbohydrates) and micronutrients (vitamins and minerals) that your machine needs.

In order to make it easier for you to know what types of food you need to consume, I'm going to tell you a little bit about them, why you need them, how to select them, and, of course, what they will help you accomplish.

## 1. PROTEINS: The Bricks of the Wall

In this chapter we're going to talk about your body as if it were a building. Believe me, it will be the easiest way to learn and remember what you're about to read.

Proteins are very important to the body because your skin, muscles, organs, and glands need them. Proteins help repair our cells and produce new ones. If you want to gain muscle and achieve a toned body, you're going to have to build more muscle cells. So, in keeping with our building metaphor: proteins are the bricks that hold the building together, and without them there is no structure.

Proteins also help with digestion, balancing hormones, and maintaining your mood. Proteins make you feel full because they take longer to digest, and they also have a greater thermic effect than carbohydrates, which means the body invests more calories in digesting them.

Proteins are made up of small units called amino acids. There are twenty types of amino acids that come together to form a brick, but we consume only nine of them through food (these nine are called essential amino acids). These are bricks we cannot manufacture; they are special, and we need to go to the hardware store to get them. The other eleven amino acids are actually manufactured in the body (they are called nonessential amino acids).

All essential amino acids are found in animal proteins, such as those derived from eggs, milk, dairy products, fish, meat, and poultry. However, plant-based proteins don't contain them all; let's just say that they are weaker bricks. On the other hand, animal proteins and derivatives have high levels of cholesterol and saturated (unhealthy) fat. This is why we can't eat unlimited amounts of animal protein—like every other food, proteins have calories and must therefore be consumed in moderation.

The best protein choices are:

▶ **Lean meats:** White meats and poultry have the same amounts and quality of protein as red meats, but red meats have more saturated fats, which are harmful to your health. If you happen to love red meat, choose a lean cut such as tenderloin or buffalo/bison. I personally prefer white meats such as chicken and turkey without the skin (roasted, parboiled, or grilled).

▶ **Fish:** They're as nutritious as meats but hold greater benefits because they contain polyunsaturated fatty acids such as omega-3s that can prevent cardiovascular diseases. Select whitefish and bluefish. Go straight to my grocery list at the end of the book, where you'll find them all.

▶ **Eggs:** An inexpensive, practical, versatile, and easy-to-digest protein. Eggs are a concentrated source of protein (over seven grams of protein per egg) and they are full of amino acids, omega-3 fatty acids, iodine, and iron. Don't worry about the yolk, since studies have shown that it has no effect on cholesterol levels, contrary to what was previously believed. Nevertheless, it's important to consume yolks in moderation—no more than one or two a day—since they do contain more calories than just the egg whites.

▶ **Low-fat dairy:** Low-fat dairy is a great source of protein, especially Greek yogurt and kefir because they also contain probiotics that improve digestion and immunity. Many people are lactose intolerant and often feel bloated or heavy when they consume dairy. This doesn't happen, however, with yogurt and kefir, as they contain almost no lactose. You should be mindful to select dairy products that have a fat content of 1 percent or lower because the whole versions are loaded with saturated fat. My favorite is 0 percent Greek yogurt, and I often substitute vegetable derivatives such as almond milk for milk and cheeses in order to avoid bloating.

▶ **Legumes and nuts:** Although legumes contain a fair amount of protein, they have less value to your body than other protein sources. I hardly ever eat them, to be honest. They don't contain all the parts we need to make a brick, and because they also contain carbohydrates, we're just going to go ahead and count legumes in the carbohydrate group. On the other hand, nuts (which I love), which also provide only incomplete proteins, also contribute healthy fatty acids, so we're going to go ahead and count them as fats.

## HOW MUCH PROTEIN DO YOU NEED?

To find out how much protein you need, you can take your weight in pounds and divide that number by two. The result is the amount (in grams) of protein that you should ideally consume each day. For example, a woman who weighs 150 pounds would need to eat 75 grams of protein daily, and a man who weighs 180 pounds would need at least 90 grams.

Practically speaking, we could say that at every meal, at least 30 percent of your plate should contain a good source of protein. This will ensure that you eat enough during the day to meet your needs, and it will also help you curb your desire to eat carbohydrates and junk food.

It's best to eat small amounts of protein throughout the day rather than a very large portion only once or twice a day, because larger portions can be difficult to digest. Eating this way also ensures that your body uses the right amount of protein, as it does not have the ability to use it all up at the same time. Remember that if you exceed your daily amount, the rest will be stored as fat or eliminated.

### 2. CARBOHYDRATES: The Energy You Need

There's no use in having a nice building if we can't turn on the lights. That energy, that "electricity," your body needs in order to function is provided by carbohydrates. Starting today, carbohydrates will be your best allies. Why? Because there is no cell in your body capable of functioning without the energy that carbohydrates provide. You need that injection of energy in order to eat, exercise, and be in a good mood. It is completely absurd to believe that carbohydrates are bad, but you have to learn to consume them in moderation.

## WHAT HAPPENS WHEN YOU EAT A CARB?

When you consume carbohydrates your body breaks them down and forms molecules that can be absorbed by the intestines. From your intestines they reach the liver, and from there they are distributed throughout the body through your bloodstream. Once they are in the blood, insulin, a hormone that is produced in the pancreas, is responsible for regulating and controlling your body's blood sugar levels.

When there is a lot of sugar in your blood because you have eaten too many carbohydrates, insulin sends your body the message to store it in your liver and muscles as glycogen. This is the body's sugar reserve for when you're not eating. But your liver and muscles can take only so much. If there is too much sugar, the excess is stored as fat. Why am I telling you all this? Because you need to know how everything works, since this is the key to understanding and selecting what will work for you.

Your body absorbs certain carbohydrates very quickly, thus spiking your blood sugar levels. Other carbohydrates take longer to be digested, and you absorb them slowly. When this happens, your blood sugar levels remain stable, which prevents insulin from telling your body to store the glycogen as fat. Needless to say, you need to go for the slow carbohydrates rather than the fast ones.

Why is your body quicker to absorb certain carbohydrates than others? It has to do with the amount of dietary fiber they contain. Fiber is the indigestible part of food, and you can find it in the outer casings of cereal seeds, in stems, in leaves, and in the skins of vegetables and fruits. Fiber brings many benefits to our gastrointestinal health, and it's super important when it comes to controlling your appetite. Fiber adds volume to your food, which makes you feel full faster. And best of all, it has no calories.

## HOW MANY CARBS DO YOU NEED?

Your activity level, body type, and fitness goals determine how many grams of carbs you should consume every day. For most active people, carbs typically represent about 40 percent of the day's calories, which usually amounts to about 150 to 200 grams of carbs per day. But the truth is, I don't think a healthy diet is about counting amounts of carbohydrates, fats, or protein—you just need to learn to select high-quality foods.

Avoid refined (or quick-absorption) carbs. These types of carbs are processed and stripped of their fiber and other nutrients. Their structure is altered, which means they enter the bloodstream as if they were an injection of sugar, which triggers the release of insulin that turns sugar into fat instead of energy. Refined carbs have been linked to diseases of the heart, kidneys, liver, and pancreas.

Here's a list of refined carbs you should try to stay away from:

▶ Refined corn, rice, and wheat used to make breads, pastas, biscuits, and pastries, for example.
▶ Juices, mashed potatoes, starches.
▶ Sugar and honey: Sugar contains no nutrients. It only makes you gain weight, contributes to tooth decay, and raises your risk of heart disease and diabetes. And although honey does

contain nutrients, it's loaded with sugar and calories. Replace sugar with stevia.

► Milk and other dairy products: Despite being rich in proteins, milk products are usually loaded with fats and sugar. A good protein choice is 0 percent Greek yogurt or kefir. Leave the milk and cheeses for cheat meal days only, once a week. Replace them with dairy-free products such as almond milk and almond milk cheese.

Go for slow carbs instead. Your main source of carbs should be vegetables. They are high in fiber, vitamins, antioxidants, and nutrients and because of the amount of fiber they contain, your body absorbs the carbohydrates slowly, keeping insulin under control. In addition to vegetables you can go for whole grains, since they have less effect on the insulin response than refined grains (white flour and breads or pasta).

The following is a list of slow carbs:

► **Rolled oats** are rich in protein, vitamins, and minerals. They may contain small amounts of gluten, so you can look for gluten-free options.
► **Brown rice** contains vitamins and minerals, and it's gluten-free. But 100 grams rack up 350 calories, so consume it in moderation.
► **Quinoa** contains healthy proteins, fats, and carbohydrates. High in vitamins, minerals, and proteins, as it provides eight of the nine essential amino acids. And it's gluten-free.
► **Whole millet** is rich in fiber, magnesium, and vitamin B, and it has an alkalizing effect, unlike other cereals, so it balances our pH and helps us compensate for the acidifying effects of a bad diet. It contains no gluten.
► **Corn** isn't something I recommend you consume on a regular basis if you want to lose weight. You can occasionally consume it in the form of fresh whole grains, popcorn, cornmeal, or tortillas made from whole grain corn.
► **Legumes** such as alfalfa, peas, beans, chickpeas, and lentils. They aren't my favorites, but they provide healthy carbohydrates, proteins, and fats. They are highly beneficial and contain essential amino acids.

- ▶ **Tubers and starchy vegetables** such as bananas, potatoes, and yucca (or cassava). They are rich in fiber, retain all their nutrients, provide you with energy, and are very versatile. I love eating them.
- ▶ **Whole fruits** are the exception to this group, since they are actually simple, fast carbohydrates if consumed in liquid form. But if you eat them whole, keeping the fiber (which is often in the skin) intact, you can count them in this group. They contain fructose, a kind of quick sugar, but the fiber in them slows down and cushions the rapid effect of sugar. They also provide your body with vitamins, minerals, and antioxidants. They contribute few calories, increase satiety, and help decrease your appetite.
- ▶ **Non-starchy vegetables** are packed with vitamins, minerals, fiber, and phytochemicals. They are so low in carbs and calories that they can be enjoyed at length. The list of non-starchy vegetables includes chard, artichokes, eggplant, broccoli, onions, brussels sprouts, cauliflower, asparagus, cucumbers, peppers, radishes, beets, cabbage, tomatoes, endive, lettuce, romaine lettuce, spinach, arugula, watercress, and carrots, among others. Vegetables are undoubtedly the best source of carbs!

## DON'T FORGET

When you don't eat carbs you feel anxious. Carbs signal to your brain that you have eaten—that you're happy and you're full. At the same time, carbs release substances that give your body a sense of well-being, which is why sweets are so tempting and comforting. But your brain can't tell the difference between a piece of cake and a sweet potato, so give it high-quality, nutritious food that will help you keep anxiety at bay.

### 3. FATS: The Furniture

Your building needs furniture to guarantee you comfort and security. And that's where fats come into play. Fats provide your body with energy and nutrients, but your body uses them mostly to help with other functions of the nervous and hormonal systems, as well as in the absorption of vitamins A, D, E, and K.

Triglycerides are how we store energy in our fatty tissue, and they are composed of three fatty acids and a glycerol, but these fatty acids can turn into cholesterol.

Triglycerides accumulate in fat tissue more easily than carbohydrates and proteins, so if you consume them in excess, you gain fat—and weight—more easily. Your body also stores the excess cholesterol in your arteries, which causes cardiovascular diseases. We all need to consume some fat, but we need to learn which ones.

| YES | WHY? | NO | WHY? |
|---|---|---|---|
| **Monounsaturated fatty acids:** extra-virgin olive oil, olives, legumes, nuts, dried fruits, avocados, and avocado oil | They lower your "bad" cholesterol (LDL) and raise your "good" cholesterol (HDL), which protects you from cardiovascular illnesses. | **Saturated fatty acids:** meat, sausages, cheese, whole dairy, margarine, butter | They raise your cholesterol. |
| **Omega-3 polyunsaturated fatty acids:** fish, nuts, soybeans, flaxseeds, and flaxseed oil | They lower your triglycerides and "bad" cholesterol (LDL). | **Trans-fatty acids:** They are used to make cookies, pastries, fast food, and fried foods. | Of all fats, these are the most harmful to your health. There is a strong relationship between trans-fat intake and increased risk of heart disease, insulin resistance, diabetes, inflammation, and damage to the inner walls of your blood vessels. Avoid them at all costs! |
| **Omega-6 polyunsaturated fatty acids:** sunflower seeds, wheat germ, sesame seeds, nuts, and corn | They lower your "bad" cholesterol (LDL) as well as your "good" (HDL). Consume them in moderation. | | |

So far, I've shown you how important the large components of your building are. I'm sure you already knew a lot of this, but sometimes we forget that our muscles aren't the only things at stake. When you decide to remodel your house, everything changes. The same thing happens when it comes to your body. If you do it right, there will be no problem. If you do it without guidance—taking your neighbor's advice, or trying a diet you read about in a magazine—things will go wrong. Believe me.

So, now we're going to talk about the small things that matter a lot.

## 4. VITAMINS AND MINERALS: The Decoration

Vitamins and minerals are micronutrients you need in small doses, but they are essential to the proper functioning of your body, especially if you exercise, and many of them work to keep your metabolism healthy. You can't see them, but you have no idea how much they do for you.

Vitamins are abundant in fresh and natural products, mainly fruits and vegetables. They are essential for your body to be able to use carbohydrates, fats, and proteins as energy sources. Without them, your machine would stop. They also help regulate your hormones, your nervous system, and blood clotting. Our body needs thirteen vitamins to grow and develop properly, and each and every one of them is important.

Minerals are essential when it comes to forming muscles—they are part of your muscle proteins, as well as other tissues, such as bones and teeth. They also work with vitamins to regulate your metabolism and your nerve impulses, and they make up some hormones. And as if that weren't enough, they aid the digestive process and help transport oxygen to your body's tissues, a particularly important function when you're exercising.

Some of the most important minerals are sodium, potassium, calcium, phosphorus, magnesium, and sulfur—these are called *macro minerals* because your body needs them in larger amounts. On the other hand, copper, iodine, iron, manganese, chromium, cobalt, zinc, and selenium are called *micro minerals* because your body needs them in smaller amounts.

I'll tell you more about minerals in the supplements chapter!

I can't close this chapter without mentioning the biggest part of your building. Do you remember how in chapter three I told you about your body composition? Since so much of it is water, it's essential to keep your body hydrated, since that's what will keep it burning.

Water is the essence of life. It's extremely important because it helps you digest what you eat; it helps your body absorb, transport, and use the nutrients it ingests; it helps eliminate your body's waste; and it helps regulate your body temperature as well as all of your metabolic functions. Without water everything stops; nothing works. Water is indispensable for our cells to breathe and stay alive. The amount of water in a person's body depends on his or her muscle mass and body-fat percentages. Generally speaking, for a man between the ages of nineteen and fifty, 50 to

60 percent of his body is water, whereas a woman in the same age range will have a slightly lower percentage, between 50 and 55 percent.

## HOW TO STAY BALANCED

Different factors, such as your metabolism, the environment, and the amount of exercise you do, will determine how much water you need, but you can generally calculate how much water you need by following this simple rule:

Drink between 25 and 50 percent of your body weight (in pounds) in ounces of water a day. That is, if you weigh 160 pounds, drink between 40 and 80 ounces of water a day. When you lose a lot of fluids, as a result of heat, physical activity, or any other reason, you become dehydrated. Dehydration impairs your performance—your body stops working properly and it accumulates waste or toxins that need to be released through proper hydration.

If you drink enough water you will avoid feeling anxious and hungry, and you'll be able to eliminate all the toxins that are at risk of causing inflammation in your body.

## HOW TO STAY HYDRATED

▶ Don't wait until you feel thirsty. Drink plenty of water throughout the day. Not only will this allow you to stay hydrated; you will also improve the appearance of your skin, protect your heart and cardiovascular system, optimize the functioning of your muscles and joints, curb food cravings, and eliminate toxins from your body.

▶ Drink water with all your meals. Avoid juices and sodas—no liquid is healthier than our vital water.

▶ Drink a large glass of water when you wake up in the morning. While you sleep, your body loses water through sweating, breathing, and its metabolic processes. It's important to replenish your body before you start the day.

▶ Bottle challenge: always carry a water bottle with you, which will mean you have no excuse not to be hydrated.

▶ Drink more while you exercise. Increase your water intake one to two hours before exercising. Drink at least 500 ounces of water, which will prepare your body for the increased activity. While you exercise take small sips totaling 4 to 8 ounces every fifteen or twenty minutes, and after training make sure you replenish your body by drinking at least 20 ounces of water.

Are you ready to get started? Keep reading to discover my secret formula to becoming your best self. Let's add some "gas to the fire"; let's burn down the building and get hot!

# 6.

# WHERE DO I BEGIN?
# BASIC ADVICE ON HOW
# TO ACHIEVE A FIT BODY

**W**elcome to your transformation!

So far I have shared my story, my motivational tools, and lots of valuable information to achieve your transformation. Now it's time to put all that knowledge to work, and that's what you're going to do today. Not tomorrow, not Monday, not next week . . . You'll start today. Because nothing is stopping you, right? I thought so.

I want to tell you how I did it. And I'll start with three basic rules that I'm sure will help you reach your destination.

## 1. 70 Percent Is Eating Healthy

Dieting to achieve a fit body is completely different from dieting to lose weight or maintain a thin body. It requires much more sacrifice and effort. That's why you have to be 100 percent determined and committed. I'm the living example of how it's possible. You don't have to punish yourself or suffer, but you will need to be consistent and determined. The first thing you need to do is define your goal: do you want to be just thin and healthy or do you want to achieve a strong, toned, and healthy body? If you're leaning toward the latter, keep reading.

There's no way around it: as long as you don't eat right, it doesn't matter how much you exercise—you're not going to see results. And I know what I'm talking about because I've been there. I used to think I could eat anything I wanted just because I exercised. The result was a flabby body with a high body-fat percentage. But when I decided to change my diet I began to notice that if I ate right while doing the same amount of exercise, sometimes even less, I got better results. By giving your body the right amount of good-quality food it deserves, you will see impressive results.

For me, eating healthy is about eating varied, sufficient, balanced, adequate, and, of course, delicious food. At times it can be hard to make healthy food choices, but here are a few easy changes you can make to achieve better results:

### ▶ Eat More Fruits and Veggies

When you eat, you shouldn't just be mindful of how many calories you consume; you also need to make sure you get the most nutrients possible. Vegetables are the greatest source of vitamins and minerals that help regulate many of the vital functions of your body. They also help prevent major diseases such as heart disease and some cancers. There's no use in achieving the perfect body if on the inside you're in a shambles.

Most people don't eat enough fruits and vegetables. If you don't have fruits and vegetables on your plate you won't feel properly satisfied, which will make you turn to high-calorie fatty and sugary foods in order to satisfy that craving. And because vegetables take up more space in your stomach, if you eat enough of them you'll feel satiated faster and with fewer calories.

Like vegetables, fruits are healthy, but you need to keep an eye on what kinds of fruit (and how many) you consume if you want to achieve a fit body. It is best to eat fruit in the morning and before or after your workouts. Later on, when we get to the meal-plan section of the book, you'll discover which fruits are my favorites and when you should eat them.

### ▶ Out with the Sugar!

Forget white sugar and sweets. Contrary to what you might think, fatty foods aren't making you fat. The main reason you're getting fat is all the sugar you eat, because it's everywhere. And remember, sugar isn't just the white stuff you see on the table . . . It wears many disguises, and it hides under names such as corn syrup, dextrose, fructose, juice concentrate, maltodextrin, raw sugar, and brown sugar. You can even find it in foods labeled as "healthy" such as fruit juice, protein bars, granolas, dressings, and so on.

Replacing all these types of sugar with a natural zero-calorie sweetener such as stevia is the best decision you can make, and your body will thank you for it.

And before you run to look it up on the Internet, let me tell you: no, your body doesn't *need* sugar. Your brain has tricked you into thinking you do. It may sound a bit radical, but if your body doesn't need sugar, why give it any? Your body needs good fuels, the kind that replenish it while giving you the energy you need: vegetables, fruits, tubers, and other carbohydrates we'll talk about later in this book.

### ▶ Beware of Whole Grains

This one might surprise you. I know that whole grain products may seem harmless, especially because we've always been told that they are a better choice than refined flour—"Choose whole wheat bread over white bread"; "Eat whole wheat pasta instead of normal pasta"— but the truth is, whole wheat bread, whole wheat pasta, whole wheat crackers, and all other things "whole" are not your friends and are far from helping you achieve the fit body of your dreams.

You'll find that we've included very few whole grain products in this book. In addition to containing fats, most of which are saturated, whole grain products have as three of their main compounds gluten, starch, and phytates—all of which can cause health problems. Gluten causes inflammation; starch quickly turns into sugar; and phytates bind to minerals, which prevents your body from absorbing the food, so in the end you're not even getting the nutrients.

It is best to replace these products with gluten-free tubers, legumes, fruits, or cereals such as brown rice, quinoa, oats (gluten-free), or natural corn. When you need to use flour in a recipe, replace it with oat bran, which is just ground oats.

### ▶ Good Fats in Moderation, Bad Fats—Never!

Many people believe that olive oil, avocados, nuts, and other "healthy" fats are harmless. That's because they focus on the benefits rather than the calories. It's not rare to see lots of fats mixed together in a single meal—a salad, for example, containing avocado, olive oil, nuts, olives, and even mayonnaise! What started out as a healthy dish is now an atomic bomb. All fats clock in at nine calories per gram, regardless of whether or not they are heart-healthy.

That's why my motto is: *Good fats, in moderation. Bad fats—never!* And by "bad fats" I'm referring to anything fried, creamy, or covered in sauces or dressings. In this book I decided not to recommend vegetable oils such as canola or corn oil because they slow down fat loss and cause inflammation. Instead, I selected good fats such as nuts, olive oil, coconut oil, or avocados, to be consumed in moderation. I also get healthy fats when I eat salmon or other "bluefishes" rich in omega-3 fatty acids.

### ▶ Quality Proteins

If you want to transform your body into a calorie-burning machine, you're going to need a lot of quality protein. As I explained earlier, proteins are the building blocks of muscle, which allows you to have an active metabolism. And as if that weren't enough, proteins are the one macronutrient that your body is least likely to store as fat!

In fact, our bodies don't just need proteins; they need amino acids. That's why you need to consume proteins that contain a wide range of amino acids such as meats, fish, and eggs. I tend to go for eggs, lean beef, buffalo or bison, pork loin, turkey, chicken, fish, and seafood. Legumes and nuts and some seeds, such as hemp and chia, also provide protein, but their quality isn't as great.

### ▶ Put a Pause on Dairy

Dairy foods are also a source of protein, but unfortunately they are loaded with fat and sugar. My recommendation is to avoid fatty cheeses, cow's milk, and its derivatives as much as possible. Vegetarian cheeses and milks are a much better alternative for your health, mainly because they contain fewer calories and no saturated fats. Almond milk and almond cheese are my favorites.

I think everyone should evaluate the effects that dairy products have on them. For example, I tolerate lactose well so I've decided to include 0 percent, sugar-free Greek yogurt in my regimen. It's a good source of protein, energy, and elements that help keep my digestive system healthy. And best of all, it helps satisfy my cravings for something sweet.

## ▶ Salt: Less Is More!

Do you want defined abs? Say goodbye to salt. Not completely, but try to keep it to a bare minimum. It's that simple. Avoid all high-sodium foods, including sausages and anything canned or processed. You'll quickly notice how your abs start to emerge. In addition to causing serious health problems, salt causes fluid retention, which makes you look heavy, swollen, and flabby.

You'll find many products labeled "no sodium" or "low sodium," and these are the best for your body. Get rid of that saltshaker! That way you won't feel tempted to use it, and believe me, once you start seeing your flat abs, you won't hesitate to replace the salt with tasty herbs and/or spices.

That said, you can't eliminate salt completely. Sodium is a necessary electrolyte for your body, but it's extremely important to balance your intake, as consuming it in excess can increase the risk of hypertension and heart attack. In general terms you should consume less than one teaspoon of salt (5 grams) a day, which is the equivalent of 2,300 milligrams of sodium. But if you suffer from hypertension or diabetes or you are fifty years old or older, you shouldn't exceed 1,500 milligrams of sodium daily (2½ grams, or half a teaspoon). However, if you sweat frequently from exercise, you can consume more than 2,300 milligrams of sodium per day. It is estimated that in one hour of exercise you can lose between one and three liters of sweat.

## 2. 20 Percent Is Exercise

I'm not going to lie to you. It is not enough to watch what you eat, and a fit body isn't built overnight. A fit body works, sweats . . . It's built on good nutrition and it's perfected with exercise. You can't have a fit body without both exercise and diet.

If you have fallen into the trap of miracle fat-burning diets, lists of foods guaranteed to give you chiseled abs, protein shakes that build your muscles . . . don't be ashamed: we've all been there. We just have to correct our mistakes and learn from them in order to get better.

The truth is, we've all been seduced—and sometimes tricked—by the promises of such miracle products, but once again, I'm going to be 100 percent honest with you: none of those products will work if you aren't willing to exercise, push yourself, and go beyond your comfort zone. If you aren't willing to do that, then you're wasting your time.

I'm not here to tell you what the best exercise is for you. There is no magic exercise to burn fat and tone your body. I can tell you what worked for me, but it won't be worth it if you're not committed to your transformation. Your body was made to burn fat; you just have to activate it daily. In order to help you stay active, I'm inviting you to download my training plans at https://www.fitplanapp.com/athletes/michelle-lewin or start training with my platform at www.lewinfitnessplatform.com, where you will find many options that can be adapted to your needs.

I once heard someone say that "hard work beats talent when talent isn't working hard enough." We are all born with different talents, and if yours is exercising, well, good for you. Your journey might be easier. But others weren't born with that talent. Yet with determination and hard work they will be able to exercise. Today I want you to commit to taking advantage of each and every one of your talents, and to start developing your ability to exercise. In these pages I'm going to share with you everything that has worked for me.

▶ **Define Your "Why"**
People tend to think that exercise is just to keep their bodies in shape and looking good. This is a big mistake. If you don't know why you're doing something, you lose sight of the benefits. Exercise is the best health insurance! In addition to helping us achieve a balanced body structure by keeping our proportions of muscle mass, body fat, bones, and organs in perfect harmony, exercise protects against heart disease, diabetes, and even cancer. It guarantees health.

That you need to eat right and exercise in order to live is a rule you must internalize and repeat to yourself every day. It needs to become a habit, like getting up every morning and brushing your teeth. So get up every day and take care of your body, your machine, your only means of transportation—your only true home.

▶ **Say No to Traditional and Boring Cardio**
Forget boring and traditional cardio. If you walk every day for forty-five minutes at the same pace and speed, you aren't going to achieve a fit body. Do you want to burn fat? The best exercise is the

one that kicks you out of your comfort zone, making you push yourself to the max by forcing you to give your very best. That's when the fun begins! It's a competition against yourself, and giving up isn't an option.

The greatest fat burning occurs when we really push ourselves. If you don't exercise regularly, you may feel restless and exhausted the first few days after you start to work out. That's normal. But after a few days, you won't feel the same and it'll start to feel easy, which means you will be burning fewer calories. Little effort, little change.

This is why it's important to ramp up your exercise routines. But how? High-intensity interval training (HIIT) is the best method. It will help you develop greater strength and speed, and it will make you better at burning fat. One of the greatest secrets to burning fat is to switch up your exercise routine as much as possible. You need to surprise your body every day.

HIIT consists of a combination of short periods of very intense cardiovascular training (at 80 to 90 percent of your maximum heart rate) and short periods of moderate or low intensity (50 to 60 percent of your maximum heart rate).

For example, if you ride a bike, you can do four minutes of moderate intensity followed by one minute of high intensity; then three minutes of low intensity, to recover energy, and then two minutes of high intensity; then finish with four minutes of low intensity and one more minute of high intensity.

▶ **Variety Is the Key**

There is no one exercise that offers all the benefits we need in a single, beautiful package, so doing a variety of exercises is your best bet if you want to see results. When you mix up your training you'll be able to develop different skills. Remember, skills are the key to success. Not just talent.

Now, here are three simple steps to integrate your exercises to achieve better results:

■ **HIIT-Type Cardio**

In order to be healthy, your body needs at least 30 minutes of cardio per day, 5 times a week, or at least 15 minutes of HIIT. But in order to lose weight and reduce your body fat, you need at least

60 minutes a day of moderate cardiovascular exercise 5 to 6 days a week, or 30 minutes daily of HIIT at least 5 days a week.

If you have never done physical activity before, start with some moderate training. After a couple of weeks you can increase the intensity and use the HIIT training method.

*Types of Exercise*
If you enjoy good health you can practice walking, cycling, spinning, swimming, using an elliptical machine, climbing stairs, hiking, paddling, skiing, climbing, or skating, among other things.

Caution: If you are overweight or out of shape, or if you suffer from injuries or other medical conditions, there are certain exercises that you shouldn't perform every day: running, tennis, paddle tennis, and squash. Try doing these on alternate days instead.

- **Strengthening Exercises**
  In order to be healthy, you need to do strength training at least two times a week. To achieve a toned and fit body you need to do strength training at least five days a week. Personally, I do strength training six times a week.

  Do two to four sets of eight to twelve repetitions for each exercise. If you don't feel you can do this just yet, start with fewer sets and gradually increase them. It's important that the last two repetitions take you to the point of muscle failure.

  *Types of Exercise*
  Exercises with weights or resistance bands, gym machines, Pilates machines, or exercise balls, among other things.

- **Stretching and Flexibility Exercises**
  Perform your stretching and flexibility exercises once you've done your cardio workout—stretching is most effective when your muscles are still warm.

  Hold each stretch for ten to thirty seconds, until you feel tightness or slight discomfort. If you want to take it to the next level, you can try yoga or tai chi classes.

► **Exercise Less**

There are people who eat very poorly and then spend four hours in the gym expecting to repair the damage caused. Less is sometimes more, especially when it comes to exercise. If you eat right, you're already 70 percent there. You just need to exercise right and for the right amount of time.

In order to leave your comfort zone you need to overcome your fears; you must be willing to experience new sensations and emotions. Instead of getting on the treadmill for sixty minutes at a moderate pace, take a chance and play around with the speed and the incline—optimize your workout and make it just thirty minutes at a much more intense pace.

If you have the time, I suggest splitting your training session. I have achieved excellent results when I've done my cardio first thing in the morning and then done my weight-training routine at night. This has given my metabolism a huge boost! My body is activated at two different times of the day, forcing my machine to burn fat.

► **Change Constantly**

Once you've been doing the same exercise for a while, your body has a tendency to adapt and stagnate. This is why you've probably noticed those people at the gym who, despite having spent a considerable amount of time working out, still look exactly the same. Many experts say that the body has the ability to adapt quickly to what we do, and I assure you, they're right. One could even say that the faster you adapt to a new routine, the higher the intensity level you need to achieve in order to burn fat.

If you find yourself in this situation and you don't feel exhausted or completely dead by the end of your gym session, it's time to make some changes. Above all, don't be afraid to pile on the weight! Oftentimes women shy away from lifting weights because they're afraid of looking like the boys. Well, I'm here to tell you that as long as you're eating right, this is literally impossible. In order to look "big" or "bulky" you need to eat meals jam-packed with carbs and calories. In order to have a slim and toned body, you need to stick to a clean and controlled diet.

# MY BEST TIPS FOR A GOOD WORKOUT ROUTINE

1. Start your workout with a warm-up (5 to 10 minutes at low intensity), followed by your cardio workouts. Then do your weight training and finish up with some stretching (5 to 10 minutes).

2. Start with moderate weight and gradually increase it. At the beginning what's most important is that you learn the proper technique to perform each exercise.

3. Perform 8 to 12 repetitions of each exercise, until your muscles feel tired. You shouldn't feel deep pain or discomfort, but you should feel some muscle fatigue.

4. Work large muscle groups (legs, chest, and back). This increases muscle mass as well as your metabolism.

5. Avoid holding your breath while performing an exercise. Exhale during the period of effort and inhale as you return to the starting position.

6. Don't overdo it. When you feel exhausted it's time to stop. If you can't perform the exercises correctly you run the risk of injury.

7. Don't lift more weight than you can handle. You can seriously injure yourself. Take it slow, and little by little you'll start to get better.

8. Don't work the same muscle group two days in a row. Give your muscles at least 24 hours' rest once you've trained them.

9. Drink enough water before, during, and after your workout session. Water is what cools down your engine; it prevents overheating and failure.

10. If you have any medical condition or previous injury, seek help from a professional trainer. Certain movements could worsen an existing injury.

## 3. Supplement Correctly and You'll Have the Remaining 10 Percent

Would you be surprised if I told you that the questions people most often ask me are, "What supplements do you take?" and "How do you take them?" instead of "What kind of diet plan do you follow?"? Well, I'm afraid it's true. People always want to find the easy way out. They want to find the magic pill, the fat burner, the miracle injection instead of choosing the discipline, effort, and sacrifice of eating right and exercising.

Here's what I have to say about that: supplements will never replace diet and exercise, but adding them can help you achieve everything your body needs. It's a fine balance. You need a bit of everything, but in the right measure.

Yes, I think supplements can be very good and useful, but above all they must be safe. I also think it's important to understand that supplements aren't going to do the work for you. Sports supplements were created for just that: sports and exercise. The labels don't say, "Go home, lie down, and wait for the results." If you do that, the results simply won't come, regardless of how much you paid for the products. So if you aren't ready for a change yet, my best advice is, don't waste your money on magic supplements. They simply don't exist.

Although there are many products that promise to improve performance during exercise, reduce body fat, improve recovery, increase muscle mass, speed up your metabolism, or help you achieve your goal faster, a number of these products may not be suitable for everyone. Your vitamin and supplement needs vary depending on your age, weight, physical condition, daily activity, and illnesses (if any), among other things. External factors such as smoking and alcohol and caffeine consumption, as well as extreme dieting and eating too many processed or unhealthy foods, can affect how you assimilate these supplements. All this is to say that it isn't enough to take good supplements in the right amounts—you need to prepare your body so it can use them properly.

Many people choose not to use supplements because they feel they get everything they need through a balanced diet. Well, to these people I say a balanced diet abundant in fresh and natural products such as fruits and vegetables will offer many necessary nutrients. However, there is no food that contains all necessary vitamins and minerals. No human being is equal to any other human being, which is why our needs vary and we need to replenish our bodies with what we lose through training, stress, intense sports, and so on.

Now, it's very important that you understand that if you don't eat balanced meals, if your food isn't fresh, if you consume large amounts of processed products, you aren't consuming food. You're filling up with products, nothing else. Food is what truly nourishes your body, and as long as you make the right choices, you will have to resort to fewer supplements. But when foods are processed, they lose all their nutritional value, leaving them loaded with pesticides and preservatives that contain very few nutrients. Now do you understand why balancing your diet is 70 percent of the effort? You would need tons and tons of supplements if they were to do the entire job for you.

Later on I will dedicate an entire chapter to telling you about what supplements I use and how I use them. But for now, I want you to remember this:

> **You'll never reap the benefits of taking supplements if you don't persevere in your commitment to healthy eating and regular exercise. No product has miraculous properties, and unless you change your lifestyle, you aren't going to see any results.**

In this chapter I've told you the three things you need know in order to reshape your habits and your life. But I also want to share with you four other things you need to do if you want to start seeing changes. If you aren't in total control of all aspects of your life, everything will be slower, the mountain will become steeper, and you will end up exhausted and defeated.

## 1. Sleep Well, Live Better

Numerous studies have proven that a lack of sleep can have terrible effects on your ability to concentrate and to process your ideas. It can alter your mood, and it can even lead to weight gain. If you don't get enough sleep you are most surely paving the way to illness.

Do you remember chapter three? (If you don't, take a break and go back to it). I told you about how important it is to check your hormones before you start this program. That's because many of the hormones I told you about perform their functions depending on how much time you spend asleep and how much time you spend awake.

The human growth hormone, for example, is affected by sleep. You can spend hours at the gym trying to build muscle, but if you aren't getting enough sleep, your body will simply not be able to build that muscle. Your muscles don't grow while you're exercising; thanks to this hormone they actually grow while you rest.

A lack of sleep also raises the body's cortisol levels. Cortisol is a hormone responsible for activating the accumulation of fat and releasing large amounts of sugar into your body. This process triggers cravings for carbohydrates and sugar. Have you noticed how you feel the morning after you've had a long night? I'm sure you've felt like eating the entire fridge, as well as the pantry, in one sitting.

To make matters worse, two other very important "hunger hormones" are related to sleep: leptin and ghrelin. Leptin suppresses your appetite and ghrelin increases it. When you don't get enough sleep, leptin levels fall and ghrelin levels increase. Consequence? You're always hungry!

Other than making sure your hormones don't fall into disarray, it's important that you get enough rest and sleep in order to have a good training session as well as a good recovery. Don't overdo it. Allow your body some time to rest and recharge. Ideally, every week you should take a day or two off from training (I take one).

When you have a clear goal in mind and you know where you're going, you need to be willing to sacrifice a few things, including your nights out partying. But believe me, it will be worth every sacrifice. It will be worth it when you arrive at the gym rested, ready to do your best, not with a swollen body and self-sabotaging anxiety. It's also important to be organized in order to plan your activities and your time off. Keep a list of the tasks and activities you need to complete so that your rest time is just as important as your next meeting.

> The road will be easier if you have the support of your family and your partner. Surround yourself with more support and less temptation; that's what will get you closer to your goal. I personally never would have been able to make it without Jimmy's help.

## 2. Control Your Anxiety to Control Your Life

You need to know your enemy if you want to defeat it. And the first step to beat your anxiety is to learn what makes you anxious. You may feel anxious due to several factors, such as a hormonal disorder, an extreme diet, dehydration, stress, feeling overwhelmed at work, or even natural reasons such as the onset of menstruation. All women have been or will go through it!

I'm sure you've felt this anxiety, probably between meals, and it usually comes in the form of an intense craving to eat sugary, high-calorie foods. It's as if there were a voice in your head telling you: Eat! Eat! Eat!

Serotonin is the substance that tells your body that you're satisfied and happy. Oftentimes when you have low serotonin levels you feel sad and depressed, which manifests itself in a greater need to eat sweets, because sweet or high-fat foods tend to generate pleasure.

**How can you increase your serotonin levels in order to curb your anxiety?**

- ▶ Eat more protein: Protein will help you balance your blood sugar and help you reduce sugar cravings.
- ▶ Eat more fiber: Fiber helps you feel fuller. Vegetables, nuts, and seeds such as chia seeds and flaxseeds are high in fiber.
- ▶ Consume less sugar: Consuming sugar will only increase your need for it. Replace all sugar with stevia and keep temptations at bay.
- ▶ Consume more tryptophan: Tryptophan is an amino acid that helps produce serotonin. It can be found in turkey, chicken, fish, eggs, sesame seeds, and squash.
- ▶ Exercise more: When you exercise you release substances called endorphins that make you happy and feel less anxious. Practicing relaxation techniques such as yoga, meditation, or tai chi is also very useful in controlling anxiety, especially if you lead a very hectic life.
- ▶ Snack more: Remember how I told you that you need to eat every three hours? Basically, it's to control anxiety. Believe me, you will feel much fuller and it will be easier to keep your portion sizes under control.
- ▶ Stress less and rest more: Stress and a lack of sleep throw your hormones off balance, which in turn alters your appetite.

### 3. Beware of Alcohol

We all know how bad alcohol is for our health!

It's one of the worst saboteurs, as it weakens your muscles, decreases your muscle mass and strength, and causes muscle pain, cramps, and fatigue.

Most alcoholic beverages are just empty calories. They have no nutrients, and all they provide you with is sugar that your body does not use and ultimately stores as fat. Alcohol also causes inflammation and dehydration, which make you feel weak, tired, and slow. And to make things worse, you'll follow it up with a great meal, because after intoxicating your body with alcohol, you will feel a huge craving to consume sugar and high-calorie foods, so it will be harder for you to control what you eat.

A glass of wine or an occasional celebratory drink with friends won't sabotage your efforts, but consuming too much alcohol can definitely make you go off track.

And last but not least . . .

### 4. A Definitive No to Cigarettes and Drugs

If you continue to smoke, no matter how much time and effort you invest in improving your body on the outside, it will soon be destroyed on the inside. Smoking damages and ages your organs—which are the indispensable parts of your engine, of your whole body. Cigarettes cause cancer and premature death, and that alone is reason enough to stop. But on top of that, smoking is closely related to being sedentary and having a poor diet. We hardly ever see people who train and watch what they eat with a cigarette in their hand. You'd have to be very silly to burn all your efforts in the few minutes a cigarette lasts.

It's worth pointing out that although alcohol and cigarettes sabotage all your efforts, the use of drugs is even worse. In addition to the serious damage they can cause to your health, they bring no benefits whatsoever. They slowly destroy your life and your body. By all means: stay away!

Your body is your home, your temple, your machine—the object that receives pleasure and care and the only space that is really yours. Don't ruin it! Treat it like a palace, not like a dump.

Are you ready? Are you feeling motivated?

Now comes the most important chapter of this book: the Hot Body Diet Plan!

Let the party begin!

# 7.

# THE HOT BODY DIET
# MEAL PLAN

**I want you to** ask yourself a few questions before we move into this chapter: How badly do you want to achieve the body of your dreams? How much are you willing to sacrifice in order to have it? Think that every moment that you hesitate, there is someone else doing the work. The minutes you spend regretting the fact that you don't have the body you want someone else is investing in eating right and training hard to get what they want.

If you aren't willing to sacrifice everything you've got, then I think you need to consider whether this is really what you want. You have to stop fooling yourself and simply accept the fact that this isn't really your goal. This is the dream of the warrior who's really ready to make a change. This is the dream of someone who isn't afraid to change, someone who is craving to try something new, to challenge herself every day.

If that's you, then welcome to my world.

Now is the time to act. You have reached the most important chapter of this book. Here you will find the secret to starting the transformation you are looking for. So far I have told you about everything that has worked for me, the changes I have experienced, and everything I have had to face on this long journey. I have had good days and days when all I wanted was to run away. But when I saw the results of my effort, when

I saw my own transformation, I knew that I had made the right decision. The best decision of my life. And nothing—I tell you, nothing—will be more satisfying than feeling good about yourself, the skin you inhabit, your body.

## A. PREPARE!

This is where your transformation starts. Here you stop being a "cow that chews on its frustrations," to become the "lioness that goes hunting." For that you must leave behind your comfort zone and get into every nook and corner of your house, your life, and even your consciousness. The advice you will find here is very practical, and I need you to stay with me. I'm with you. Open your mind and you will find things that you didn't know you had, and I'm not just talking about your pantry. You'll see!

We're going to start with the three most important places on your path to transformation. I don't want you to read; I want you to act. I want you to put everything I tell you into practice, step-by-step. By the time you reach the end of this chapter, I can guarantee your life will have taken a 180-degree turn.

### THE KITCHEN

1. Prepare and season your foods with Himalayan sea salt, pepper, garlic, onion, parsley, oregano, coriander, thyme, rosemary, ginger, basil, curry, cumin, mustard, olive oil, balsamic vinegar, and lemon.
2. Avoid processed sauces and dressings. Everything that comes in a bottle, can, or package needs tons of additives for preservation, including salts and other chemicals that cause fluid retention and inflammation. The more natural, the better!
3. Bye-bye, frying pan. Cook your food in a Teflon-coated pan, in a wok, or in the oven in order to minimize the amount of oil you use.
4. Eat lots of raw vegetables. These will help you feel full and keep your anxiety at bay. Avoid excessive cooking—the fresher they are, the more nutrients they carry.

5. Eat several times a day. If you skip breakfast, if you don't snack, or if you have a quick and tiny lunch, you'll feel hungry at the end of the day. It will be difficult to control your appetite and you will eat the entire contents of your refrigerator.

6. Eat enough protein and carbohydrates. These will keep you satisfied and active and you won't feel so hungry during the day.

7. Use less salt and stay away from artificial sweeteners. Salt causes fluid retention and causes your body to absorb more glucose (sugar) in the intestine. Don't use more than half a teaspoon per day, and use stevia instead of artificial sweeteners (stick to no more than two sachets a day).

8. Drink two to three liters of water a day. Don't wait until you feel thirsty, since thirst is a sign that your body is already dehydrated.

9. Remove all temptations from your home. Also, don't make up excuses by saying, "It's for when I have guests over" or "It's for my children." If there's something you want your children to eat, then take them to a place where they can enjoy it and make a celebration out of it. But not at home!

10. Make a grocery list. Buy only what you need. You'll find my grocery list at the end of the book. Don't go shopping when you're hungry, and never even think about buying something "for later."

## THE GYM

1. Don't train when you're hungry. If you do not have the energy to perform an activity, that means you haven't eaten enough during the day or you've skipped your pre-workout snack. Make sure you eat three main meals (breakfast, lunch, and dinner), and have a small snack thirty minutes before you work out; it can be a fruit smoothie or a piece of fruit.

2. Beware of energy drinks. They contain lots of caffeine and sugar. You'll feel energized, but in the long run they will make it harder and harder for you to see results. Choose calorie-free energy options such as green tea.

3. Avoid fake energizers. Eating sweets or other sugary foods before training can give you a burst of energy, but then due to a phenomenon called reactive hypoglycemia, they quickly deplete you before you're done exercising.

4. Exercise five to six times a week. A good routine should include weight training (forty-five minutes) and cardiovascular exercises (forty-five minutes) in order to burn more calories and lose fat effectively. Rest for a day or two before resuming your training.

5. Follow your workout routine. Don't just plan it. If you decide to exercise five days a week, stick to it. Writing it down and not doing it won't burn calories. Whether there's rain, thunder, or lightning, you have to show up to fulfill your commitment.

6. Wear appropriate clothing and use the right equipment. Don't wear overly tight clothing, as it prevents natural perspiration. Don't wear waterproof clothing. Make sure your accessories are in good shape (especially your sneakers). Also, it's important to look good in order to feel good while you train. You're not just training your body; you're training your mind.

## ORGANIZE YOUR LIFE

1. Avoid cigarettes, alcohol, and drugs that can make you feel weak or tired, alter your coordination, and reduce alertness, making you prone to injury. If you want to see results, stay away.

2. Get enough rest. You need more than six hours of sleep at night. Remember that sleep gives you mental health and physical strength, reduces anxiety levels, stimulates the growth of your muscles, keeps your hormones balanced, and helps you burn more fat.

3. Choose five bad habits and change them. It takes time to adopt new behaviors. For every bad habit you quit, such as drinking alcohol or soft drinks, create a new habit, like drinking more water. Try it, practice it, and make it a habit.

4. Don't accept, without thinking, all the advice you receive. Not everyone is an expert. The advice of those who have learned to do something on their own may not be appropriate for you.

Advice can help, but there is nothing better than getting an expert opinion. TV advertising or what the Internet has to say about a certain product is most certainly the worst advice you can get.

5. Don't despair. As I said earlier, this is a marathon, not a sprint. You will see results to the extent that you stick to what you've promised yourself and what you've planned. Don't look for shortcuts. Don't invest in "supplements" or miracle preparations. Everything will come, as long as you persevere.

6. Consult with a professional. If you are concerned that your weight isn't improving despite good nutrition and exercise, talk to your doctor or a nutritionist who can evaluate your situation and guide you in the right direction. There might be a health problem that's interfering with your results, or it might just be that the portions you are eating aren't what your body needs.

7. Don't leave anything for tomorrow. Just as you can't leave taking a bath or brushing your teeth for the next day, you can't leave your food and exercise for tomorrow. Your health can't wait.

8. Don't let yourself down. Don't fool yourself. Don't give up. Do your best; push yourself to the max; don't make excuses or sit around waiting for others. Start with what little you have, and I can guarantee that you'll achieve great results. And those results will be the greatest reward!

## B. GET READY!

Once you're done with all the tasks I gave you in the last section, then you're ready to move forward. I want you to imagine that you're in the middle of the race and people are encouraging you: Don't stop! Keep going! In this section we'll take a moment to look at what you're going to eat, because I want you to know and have everything you need in order to achieve your goals.

Write down and repeat the five rules you're going to live by over the course of the next twenty-eight days.

## FIRST: I WILL SELECT GOOD FOODS 70 PERCENT OF THE TIME

From now on these will be your lines of action; this is what you will say to yourself with passion and firmness:

- I will eat more fresh fruits and veggies.
- I will get rid of sugar and any food that contains it.
- I will allow only whole products to enter my home.
- I will eat only good fats, in moderation.
- I will choose quality proteins.
- I will put a pause on dairy.
- I will banish the salt from my kitchen.

In chapter six, I told you how I learned to eat this way and how it has worked for me. If you think you aren't ready to do this yet, go back and take the time to read that chapter again.

| WHAT FOODS SHOULD YOU EAT? | WHAT FOODS SHOULD YOU STAY AWAY FROM 90 PERCENT OF THE TIME? |
| --- | --- |
| Homemade popcorn without oil or salt; rice crackers or gluten-free corn. | Cookies, cakes, pastries, and desserts with saturated fats and sugar. |
| Avocado, olive, and coconut oil; homemade peanut butter, natural nuts, and almond flour. | Corn, canola, sunflower, soy, or mixed vegetable oil; sour cream, butter, margarine, mayonnaise, high-fat creams, processed peanut butter, canned nuts, and peanuts covered with caramel or spices. |
| Sugar-free Greek yogurt, almond milk or another vegetable milk, vegetarian cheeses (almond). | Whole milk and yogurt; cheese: cheddar, Muenster, hard white, American, Brie, cream, Gouda, Gruyère. |
| Greek yogurt ice cream, pudding, or flan made with almond milk or another vegetable milk. | Ice cream, milkshakes, puddings, or flans made with whole milk. |
| Light gelatin and protein drinks. | Sweets and goodies made with fat and sugar. |
| Dark cocoa powder and 70 percent dark chocolate without sugar. | Milk chocolates with added sugar. |
| Lean meat cuts (tenderloin, pork loin, bison or buffalo meat), bluefish, chicken breast, low-fat turkey breast. | Ribs, canned meat, pork bacon, ham, chorizo, fried chicken with skin, sausage, bacon or sliced salami (deli type), bologna, and mortadella. |

| WHAT FOODS SHOULD YOU EAT? | WHAT FOODS SHOULD YOU STAY AWAY FROM 90 PERCENT OF THE TIME? |
|---|---|
| Low-fat egg whites, cooked. Just one yolk per day. | Eggs fried in oil or butter. |
| Protein pancakes and muffins. | Sweet granola, pancakes (from pancake mix), packaged sugar-free muffins. |
| Oatmal or oat bran. | Processed flour, white bread, croissants. |
| Brown rice, quinoa, and legumes such as red beans, black beans, lentils, etc. | White rice, fried rice, rice cooked with margarine or butter, pastas with cream sauce, and packaged rices and noodles. |
| Fresh whole fruits. | Natural fruit juices or canned fruit. |
| Sweet potatoes, yucca, plantains, baked sweet potato, yucca or plantain chips, fresh or roasted vegetables. | French fries, potato gratin or potatoes with cream, fried vegetables served with mayonnaise. |
| Water, flavored water, and natural infusions such as green tea, hibiscus tea, black tea, etc. | Sodas, bottled or sweet juices. |
| Natural herbs and spices. | High-sodium seasonings or bouillon cubes. |

## SECOND: PORTION SIZE DOES MATTER

When you can't measure, weigh, or know exactly how much you can eat of a certain food, you oftentimes end up eating more than you should, and even if you're eating very healthy food, this may be that "pebble in the shoe" that doesn't allow you to reach your goal. The secret is to learn a simple and practical way to measure the amount of food you need to eat.

In the twenty-eight-day plan we've prepared for you, you'll find the recommended portion size for each meal, according to the caloric plan that's meant for you (1,200, 1,500, and 1,800 calories). You need to stick to those portions. Because even though all these recipes are very healthy, everything (except water) contains calories, and if you eat too much it can become hard for you to lose weight and see the body changes you are looking for. Even though I've already met my weight goal and I train and eat carefully simply to stay in shape, I keep an eye on portion sizes for all my meals.

That is why I recommend buying an electronic food scale—it's a good way to familiarize yourself with the size and portions of your meals. Weigh your food once you've cooked it and put it on your plate. Look at the space it occupies and how it looks. That way next time you don't know how much you need to eat of a certain food when you're away from your scale, you can try to visualize that mental picture. Remember what you have practiced, and stick to it. Don't feel you need to eat it all! Do not overeat! It's okay to eat just what your body needs and leave the rest on the plate.

## Watch Out! Light Products Are the Kings of Deception.

Many people confuse *light* with *harmless*. What they don't know is that for a product to be considered "light" all it needs is to contain a third fewer calories or 50 percent less fat than the regular version. *Light* is therefore not synonymous with *healthy*, nor does it mean that it is low in calories. All it indicates is that it contains fewer calories than another similar product. Consume it with great caution! And always respect the recommended serving.

### THIRD: LESS IS MORE!

The most important part of this plan is that you enjoy every bite. If you start a highly restrictive meal plan that steals the aroma and flavor away from your dishes, you'll probably end up getting bored. When we don't enjoy what we eat, it's easier to give up. Eating well is not synonymous with torture. You just have to learn to select the healthier versions of the foods you love most.

It's also easier when you start out with quality ingredients. Everything tastes better when it's fresh, and if you have the opportunity to cook every day, even better. But if you're strapped for time, there's always the option of making easy preparations (grilled, baked, wok) and storing them in the refrigerator or the freezer. You could also reserve one day a week to prepare all your meals so all you have to do every day is heat them up and eat them.

You don't need to be a chef to eat right. With basic knowledge and a little creativity you can eat delicious, healthy food. I encourage you to take a look at my grocery list, where you will find a variety of herbs and spices than can be very handy when it comes to adding flavor, color, and variety to your dishes.

> Buy fresh fruits and veggies; they are naturally tastier. Enjoy their variety of flavors without having to add many condiments.

## FOURTH: HAVE A CHEAT MEAL ONCE A WEEK

You can have a cheat meal once a week by selecting foods that aren't a part of this meal plan. In addition to the 150 meals I suggest you eat over the course of the next twenty-eight days in order to achieve the body you want, I recommend you give yourself a weekly "cheat meal" starting during week three. The idea is that you introduce it once you're familiar with and focused on your plan. This will make it a lot easier for you to pick up the plan where you left it.

> If you eat right 90 percent of the time, it doesn't matter if your meals aren't ideal the other 10 percent of the time!

You can use your cheat meal when you're feeling stuck in a rut or you're craving a particular food (I used to eat bread, chips, and cheese-cake, which is my favorite dessert). In fact, the cheat meal is a great metabolic accelerator: since it gives your body something it wasn't expecting, it's as if you added gas to the fire. Your body will feel rewarded, and you'll trick it into believing that the time has come to release all that fat it's been reserving for those "bad times" when it thinks it might need it.

But be careful! If you don't eat healthily most of the time and if you don't do your regular exercise, the cheat meal simply doesn't make sense.

## FIFTH: STAY HYDRATED

Water is the essence of life. It allows our bodies to perform their functions. It cools down our engine. If the engine is damaged, the car stops. It's important to consume two to three liters of water a day to replenish what you lose. In chapter five I talked about the importance of staying hydrated.

And remember: never wait to feel thirsty—when that happens you're already dehydrated. Make it a habit always to carry a water bottle with you. That guarantees that there will be no excuses, and carrying a water bottle is a way of reminding yourself to drink. Always choose water—no drink can replace the benefits of consuming natural water. It contains no calories, sugars, coloring, or added substances.

## Here Are My Basic Rules for Getting Started

1. Make the decision and start today.
2. In order to stay focused, write down your list of reasons.
3. Don't set impossible goals. Consult your doctor or nutritionist.
4. Visit your doctor to make sure you're in good health.
5. Keep a food diary and write down everything you eat.
6. Fill out the forms you will find at the end of the book. Use them to record your measurements and keep track of your daily supplements, as well as the exercises performed and the calories burned per day.
7. Take a selfie wearing sports clothes or a bathing suit. You'll be amazed when you start to see the changes, and that will help keep you motivated.
8. Remove all forbidden foods from your fridge and pantry. Everything!
9. Plan your meals. You can set aside a day or two to plan out and prepare the food you'll eat for the rest of the week.
10. Don't obsess over eating right every day. Instead, make sure that by the end of the week you have achieved 90 percent of your goals.
11. Stay as active as you can. Don't sit for more than three hours in a row. Climb stairs, walk, get up from the chair to look for something, but also devote at least one hour of your day to exercise.
12. Don't focus on results. Take it one day at a time: "Just for today I'm going to eat healthily, I'm going to keep my portions under control, and I will exercise."
13. Do not fall into the trap of miracle pills, "fat-burning" injections, or commercial supplements that promise magical changes in thirty days.

14. Be patient. You didn't gain weight overnight. Losing between 1.1 and 2.2 pounds per week is perfectly fine and healthy.
15. Enjoy the journey and achieve a fit body, without becoming obsessed.

# C. TAKE ACTION!

The time has come. I trust that you have done everything in your power to get organized, plan, and take action. You're here, standing in front of your goal, and now you're just a whistle blow away from starting the race. We'll begin with a plan, designed especially for you, that varies in nutrients and calories. And next I will teach you how to select which plan is most suitable for your body. This is the most important step.

Calculator, pencil, and paper in hand! Let's start.

The first thing we need to do is calculate how many calories your body burns when at rest (your basal metabolic rate), and then tweak your number depending on a series of factors and your objectives.

**STEP 1: THE GENDER FACTOR**

Because this book is aimed at women, we will include the calculation for only this gender. If you happen to be a man, bear in mind that your number will be between 25 and 27.

> Multiply your weight (in kilograms) by 23. If you know your weight only in pounds, divide it by 2.2 to get it in kilos.
>
> Example: If you weigh 176 pounds, divide that number by 2.2 and you get a result of 80 kilograms. Multiply the total by 23.
>
> 80 x 23 = 1,840.

**STEP 2: THE AGE FACTOR**

- If you are under 18 years old, add 300 to the number above.
- If you are between 18 and 45 years old, leave the number as is.
- If you are between 46 and 55 years old, subtract 100 from the number above.

- If you are between 56 and 65 years old, subtract 200 from the number above.
- If you are between 66 and 75 years old, subtract 300 from the number above.

Following the same example, suppose you are between 46 and 55 years of age; then you must subtract 100 from the number above:
1,840 - 100 = 1,740

## STEP 3: THE PHYSICAL ACTIVITY FACTOR

- **No physical activity** (very sedentary life, no exercise): leave the number as it is.
- **Light physical activity** (at least 20 minutes of physical activity, whether it's tidying up around the house, doing work that requires some physical effort, walking to work): add 100 to the number above.
- **Moderate physical activity** (work that involves a considerable amount of physical effort, such as gardening or masonry, exercise, or walking 30 to 45 minutes or completing 10 thousand steps a day at a moderate pace): add 200 calories to the number above.
- **Intense physical activity** (going to the gym for at least 60 minutes every day, doing sports on a daily basis, keeping active for the rest of the day): add 300 to the number above.

Following the example above, suppose that you have a moderate level of physical activity; then you have to add 200 to the number above:
1,740 + 200 = 1,940

## STEP 4: DEFINE YOUR PURPOSE

- **Do you want to maintain your current weight?** Leave the number as it is. This value represents the calories you need to consume daily to maintain your weight.
- **Do you want to lose weight?** Subtract between 300 and 500 (calories) from the number above. These are the calories you need to subtract in order to lose one to two pounds a week.

► **Do you want to gain weight, increasing your muscle mass?**
Add 300 to 500 (calories) to the number above. This is how many calories you need to add in order to gain one to two pounds a week.

Following the example above: suppose you want to lose weight, so you'll have to subtract 500 from the previous result. That is:
1,940 - 500 = 1,440

## STEP 5: CALCULATE YOUR TOTAL DAILY CALORIES

Enter your total here: _____

Below you'll find a meal plan with suggested servings per meal or preparation based on the caloric and macronutrient distribution of a 1,200-, a 1,500-, and an 1,800-calorie plan. If your result doesn't fit exactly into one of these three scenarios, round your number of daily calories up or down to the nearest number, depending on whether you want to lose, gain, or maintain your weight. This will be your suggested serving size over the next twenty-eight days.

In our example we obtained a result of 1,440. In this case, you could follow the 1,500-calorie plan in order to lose weight, although we recommend that you increase your exercise program slightly. Another option would be to stick to the same amount of physical activity but follow the 1,200-calorie plan, which will allow you to get faster results.

We're working on you, so be mindful of your answers, analyze the situation, and commit yourself to this program that will rebuild your body and your life. Now that you know the numbers, you can move forward. And remember: to persevere is to win.

## BEFORE WE GET INTO THE RECIPES

On the following pages you will find your meal charts for every week; they contain what you need to eat every day and at every meal. Each week will have a different goal. You can substitute meals belonging to the same week, but don't switch them up if they belong to different weeks. For example, if you don't have the ingredients you need to make the suggested lunch for Day 1, you can make the lunch recipe from Day

2, because they're both from the same week. After the recipe section (page 244) you'll find a list of possible substitutions for each ingredient, which will allow you to stick to this plan over time, without ever getting bored.

Some of these recipes are very simple, and others are more complicated or may take longer to prepare; we ask that you marinate certain meats for four to eight hours with ingredients that don't add a considerable amount of calories but do add many nutrients and flavor. If you don't have all the ingredients to prepare a certain recipe, try to make it with fewer ingredients. If you don't have time to marinate some of the meats, you can try eating them without marinating them—even if that means they won't be as flavorful. Later on, when you have more time, you can prepare them and taste them as they're meant to be.

We start every week off with the Superstar Recipe of the Week, which is a recipe we're particularly fond of due to the many nutrients it contains and its versatility when it comes to preparation. These Superstar Recipes appear on different occasions throughout the plan, so when you see one you need to go back to the page where it appears for the first time.

It's very important that you have a small kitchen scale to weigh the amounts that are given in ounces, even if you're used to just estimating.

The first meal of the day is what I call a pre-workout snack, which you can eat between thirty and sixty minutes before doing your cardio. If you aren't going to start your day off with a cardio workout and you'd rather have breakfast early, you can do so and turn your pre-workout snack into a midmorning snack.

If you don't have enough time to prepare everything we give you below, you can always substitute a suggested snack with a serving of fruit (red fruit, apple, pear, mandarin, plum, peach, pineapple, etc.), four ounces of protein (fish, chicken, turkey, bison, eggs, etc.), or a whey protein shake made with water.

# WEEK 1: JUMP-START WITH JOY

| TIME | MEALS | DAY 1 | DAY 2 | DAY 3 | DAY 4 | DAY 5 | DAY 6 | DAY 7 |
|---|---|---|---|---|---|---|---|---|
| 6:00 a.m. / 7:00 a.m. | MEAL 1: PRE-WORKOUT SNACK | Egg whites + detox smoothie | Egg whites + detox smoothie | Egg whites + detox smoothie | Egg whites + detox smoothie | Egg whites + detox smoothie | Egg whites + detox smoothie | Egg whites + detox smoothie |
| 8:00 a.m. / 9:00 a.m. | MEAL 2: BREAKFAST | Oatmeal protein drink with strawberries | Spinach crepe filled with turkey and mushrooms | Oatmeal protein waffles | Oatmeal arepa + scrambled eggs | Chocolate almond oatmeal drink | Egg muffins + high-fiber whole wheat toast | Vanilla cranberry protein pancakes |
| 11:00 a.m. / 12:00 p.m. | MEAL 3: LUNCH | Buffalo tenderloin + sweet potato puree + steamed green beans | Chicken kebab + quinoa tabbouleh | Pineapple shrimp kebabs + baked sweet potato + green salad | Chicken quinoa salad bowl | Grilled salmon + sweet potato chips + grilled asparagus | Baked chicken thighs + quinoa + green salad | Red tuna, wakame, quinoa salad |
| 2:00 p.m. / 3:00 p.m. | MEAL 4: SNACK P.M. 1 | Hard-boiled egg nests with chicken and avocado | Green tea fit protein cupcake | Cucumber wheels + tuna avocado tartare | Strawberry protein pancakes | Unsalted nuts | Chocolate protein donut | Popcorn |
| 5:00 p.m. / 6:00 p.m. | MEAL 5: DINNER | Zucchini tortillas + salmon tartare | Asian chicken cabbage wraps | Tandoori chicken + Greek salad | Grilled buffalo ribeye + pico de gallo | Asian chicken salad + Asian vinaigrette | Fish papillote + julienned vegetables | Turkey stew + mixed salad |
| 8:00 p.m. / 9:00 p.m. | MEAL 6: SNACK P.M. 2 (IF YOU'RE HUNGRY) | Marbled fit protein cupcake | Peanut butter chocolate protein shake | Chocolate protein pancakes | Peanut butter chocolate protein balls | Artichoke and lemon dip | Chicken spinach burger | Turkey asparagus rolls |

## WEEK 2: MOTIVATION AND ENERGY

| TIME | MEALS | DAY 8 | DAY 9 | DAY 10 | DAY 11 | DAY 12 | DAY 13 | DAY 14 |
|---|---|---|---|---|---|---|---|---|
| 6:00 a.m. / 7:00 a.m. | MEAL 1: PRE-WORKOUT SNACK | Egg whites + apple green tea infusion | Egg whites + apple green tea infusion | Egg whites + apple green tea infusion | Egg whites + apple green tea infusion | Egg whites + apple green tea infusion | Egg whites + apple green tea infusion | Egg whites + apple green tea infusion |
| 8:00 a.m. / 9:00 a.m. | MEAL 2: BREAKFAST | Quinoa arepa + tomato scrambled eggs | Tuna yucca fritters | Green plantain turkey empanadas | Sweet potato tuna croquettes | Spanish tortilla + criollo potatoes | Chicken-and-avocado-filled yucca arepas | Baked sweet potato boats stuffed with turkey and vegetarian cheese |
| 11:00 a.m. / 12:00 p.m. | MEAL 3: LUNCH | Baked potato stuffed with chicken chili + green salad | Buffalo fajitas + brown rice + steamed broccoli | Crispy fish sticks + baked yucca fries + pico de gallo | Chicken curry + brown rice + mixed salad | Grilled pork loin + brown rice + steamed broccoli | Chicken breast + baked sweet potato fries + grilled vegetable kebabs | Beef tenderloin kebabs + baked criollo potatoes + pineapple-coleslaw salad |
| 2:00 p.m. / 3:00 p.m. | MEAL 4: SNACK PM 1 | Pineapple fit protein cupcake | Tzatziki + carrot sticks | Peanut butter blondies | Turkey, tomato, and lettuce sandwich | Oatmeal protein cookies | Strawberry protein shake | Protein Greek yogurt with berries |
| 5:00 p.m. / 6:00 p.m. | MEAL 5: DINNER | Chicken-stuffed portobello mushroom + pico de gallo | Chicken chili-stuffed tomatoes + vegetarian cheese | Turkey meatballs with tomato ragout + zucchini noodles | Stuffed squid + grilled asparagus | Whitefish ceviche | Tuna, avocado, cucumber, and wakame roll + ponzu sauce | Zucchini cannelloni + turkey ragout |
| 8:00 p.m. / 9:00 p.m. | MEAL 6: SNACK P.M. 2 (IF YOU'RE HUNGRY) | Lettuce turkey rolls | Light blackberry gelatin | Hot cocoa with almond milk | Vanilla protein pancakes | Turkey stew with spinach and carrots | Pistachio fit protein cupcake | Kiwi or berries with fat-free whipped cream |

# WEEK 3: DISCIPLINE AND CONSISTENCY

| TIME | MEALS | DAY 15 | DAY 16 | DAY 17 | DAY 18 | DAY 19 | DAY 20 | DAY 21 |
|------|-------|--------|--------|--------|--------|--------|--------|--------|
| 6:00 a.m. / 7:00 a.m. | MEAL 1: PRE-WORKOUT SNACK | Egg whites + antioxidant smoothie | Egg whites + antioxidant smoothie | Egg whites + antioxidant smoothie | Egg whites + antioxidant smoothie | Egg whites + antioxidant smoothie | Egg whites + antioxidant smoothie | Egg whites + antioxidant smoothie |
| 8:00 a.m. / 9:00 a.m. | MEAL 2: BREAKFAST | Walnut raisin protein waffles | Smoked salmon muffins + sweet potato and beet chips | Carrot protein pancakes | Vegetable egg white omelette + sweet potato hash browns | Cinnamon protein waffles | Egg and vegetable pizza + sweet potato cubes | Chia protein pancakes |
| 11:00 a.m. / 12:00 p.m. | MEAL 3: LUNCH | Baked pork loin + Waldorf salad | Pepper steak + baked yucca chips + mixed salad | Baked chicken + pumpkin puree + green salad | Grilled salmon, arugula, and pomegranate salad | Greek salad with chicken and nonfat feta cheese | Grilled steak + grilled vegetables + *guasacaca* | Lemon grilled fish + sweet potato puree + pineapple-coleslaw salad |
| 2:00 p.m. / 3:00 p.m. | MEAL 4: SNACK P.M. 1 | Chocolate fudge fit protein cupcake | Chicken, cucumber, and tomato salad with lemon | Almond cinnamon protein Greek yogurt | Green apple or pear + peanut butter | Turkey and mushroom scrambled eggs | Walnut raisin fit protein cupcake | Unsalted nuts |
| 5:00 p.m. / 6:00 p.m. | MEAL 5: DINNER | Chicken and vegetable noodle ramen soup | Turkey portobello burger | Curry shrimp and grilled vegetable kebabs | Seafood and stir-fried vegetable soup | Tuna lettuce wraps + pico de gallo | Fish and vegetable soup | Cheat meal |
| 8:00 p.m. / 9:00 p.m. | MEAL 6: SNACK P.M. 2 (IF YOU'RE HUNGRY) | Baked pork loin | Apple cinnamon protein shake | Avocado lemon egg salad | Banana walnut fit protein cupcake | Greek yogurt blueberry shake | Tuna stew | Pineapple light gelatin |

## WEEK 4: CELEBRATION AND REWARD

| TIME | MEALS | DAY 22 | DAY 23 | DAY 24 | DAY 25 | DAY 26 | DAY 27 | DAY 28 |
|---|---|---|---|---|---|---|---|---|
| 6:00 a.m. / 7:00 a.m. | MEAL 1: PRE-WORKOUT SNACK | Egg whites + pineapple skin infusion | Egg whites + pineapple skin infusion | Egg whites + pineapple skin infusion | Egg whites + pineapple skin infusion | Egg whites + pineapple skin infusion | Egg whites + pineapple skin infusion | Egg whites + pineapple skin infusion |
| 8:00 a.m. / 9:00 a.m. | MEAL 2: BREAKFAST | Baked eggs in stuffed peppers | Bison and pumpkin burger | Spinach and vegetarian cheese omelette with whole wheat toast | Chocolate chip fit protein waffles | Turkey and sun-dried tomato omelette + yucca chips | Smoked salmon and avocado on whole wheat toast | Egg and avocado on brown rice crackers |
| 11:00 a.m. / 12:00 p.m. | MEAL 3: LUNCH | Thai chicken vegetable stir-fry | Fish in sesame sauce + fattoush salad | Grilled sirloin steak + mixed salad with avocado | Vegetarian cheese, tomato, and arugula cauliflower pizza | Grilled chicken with lemon and sesame cream + vegetable stir-fry | Turkey stew + mixed salad with avocado | Grilled chicken with sweet-and-sour mustard + pineapple-coleslaw salad |
| 2:00 p.m. / 3:00 p.m. | MEAL 4: SNACK P.M. 1 | Artichoke and spinach hummus + carrot sticks | Apple cinnamon fit protein cupcake | Popcorn with turmeric and pepper | Blackberry protein ice cream | Turkey, arugula, and tomato eggplant rolls | Coconut fit protein cupcake | Green apple or pear + peanut butter |
| 5:00 p.m. / 6:00 p.m. | MEAL 5: DINNER | Asian chicken salad + Asian vinaigrette | Chicken chili lettuce wraps + pico de gallo | Steamed fish with ginger + grilled asparagus | Chicken vegetable stir-fry | Turkey stew + green salad | Sautéed shrimp on zucchini noodles | Cheat meal |
| 8:00 pm / 9:00 pm | MEAL 6: SNACK P.M. 2 (IF YOU'RE HUNGRY) | Strawberry protein pancakes | Green apple-smoked salmon rolls | Carrot fit protein cupcake | Turkey breast zucchini rolls | Chocolate chip fit protein cupcake | Chicken stew + eggplant chips | Chocolate protein ice cream |

# THE HOT BODY
## DIET PLAN
# menus

# fit protein cupcakes

### INGREDIENTS

3 egg whites
½ cup stevia-based sweetener
½ tsp lemon zest
3 egg yolks
1 tsp vanilla
juice of ½ lemon
2 cups almond flour
⅔ cup almond milk
1 scoop of vanilla whey protein (30 g)
1 tsp baking powder
vegetable oil spray

### INSTRUCTIONS

**1.** Preheat oven to 350°F. In a bowl and with the help of an electric mixer, beat the egg whites until they form soft peaks, about 2 minutes.

**2.** Add the sweetener and the lemon zest, and mix for 1 minute.

**3.** Add the egg yolks, vanilla, and lemon juice and continue to mix.

**4.** Add the almond flour, almond milk, vanilla whey protein, and baking powder.

**5.** Lightly spray a muffin pan with vegetable oil (you can also use baking cups), and add the mixture until completely covered.

**6.** Bake for 25 to 30 minutes. Let cool, unmold, and serve.

YIELD: 10 cupcakes (2½ oz each)

### Make These Cupcakes in 14 Different Flavors!

You can use the same basic recipe to create several different flavors. Add all quantities below to the portion of mixture needed to make *one* cupcake.

- **Marbled cupcake:** Fill ¾ of the baking cup parts with the vanilla base mixture. Take a portion equivalent to the remaining ¼ and mix it with ½ teaspoon unsweetened cocoa powder. Add the cocoa mixture to the vanilla and mix to create a marbled texture.
- **Red berries:** Add 1 tablespoon red berries (blueberries, strawberries, or blackberries).
- **Green tea:** Add 1 teaspoon matcha green tea powder.
- **Carrot:** Add 1 tablespoon grated carrots, ½ teaspoon cinnamon, ¼ teaspoon cloves, and a pinch of nutmeg.
- **Nuts and raisins:** Add 1 tablespoon chopped nuts and 1 teaspoon raisins.
- **Apple and cinnamon:** Add 1 tablespoon diced apples (keep the skin) and ½ teaspoon cinnamon.
- **Chocolate chips:** Add 1 tablespoon sugar-free chocolate chips.
- **Pumpkin:** Add 1 tablespoon pumpkin puree.
- **Chocolate fudge:** Add 1 teaspoon cocoa powder, 1 tablespoon unsweetened chocolate chips, and 1 teaspoon almond milk.
- **Coconut:** Add 1 tablespoon grated coconut (sugar-free) and a few drops of coconut essence.
- **Pistachios:** Add 1 tablespoon chopped pistachios.
- **Banana and walnuts:** Add 1 tablespoon banana puree and 1 tablespoon finely chopped walnuts.
- **Pineapple:** Add 1 tablespoon chopped pineapple and a pinch of cinnamon to taste.
- **Turmeric:** Add ½ teaspoon turmeric powder.

## DAILY MENUS

### *Day 1*

Nothing is impossible. Remove the word *impossible* from your life. As long as you're alive, you always have the power to achieve what you want. Tap into your inner strength, work hard, and be disciplined. If you truly desire something with passion, you will achieve it.

## MEAL 1: PRE-WORKOUT SNACK:

**Egg Whites + Detox Smoothie**

# egg whites

You can choose either to boil the eggs in water and eat *only the whites*, or to make an egg white scramble with any vegetable you want.

| 1,200-CALORIE PLAN | 1,500-CALORIE PLAN | 1,800-CALORIE PLAN |
|---|---|---|
| ▶ 2 egg whites | ▶ 3 egg whites | ▶ 5 egg whites |

# detox smoothie

**INGREDIENTS**

1 slice of pineapple, frozen, in pieces
½ cucumber, small
½ cup fresh spinach
1 bunch of parsley, small
1 piece of ginger, peeled
juice of 1 lemon
1 cup water
1 tbsp chia seeds
1 tbsp flaxseeds
2 stevia packets
ice

**INSTRUCTIONS**

1. Put all ingredients in a blender and mix for 1 minute.
2. Serve and enjoy.

**YIELD: 1½ cups (16 oz)**

| 1,200-CALORIE PLAN | 1,500-CALORIE PLAN | 1,800-CALORIE PLAN |
|---|---|---|
| ▶ 8 oz | ▶ 12 oz | ▶ 16 oz |

**DAY 1**

## MEAL 2: BREAKFAST:
### Oatmeal Protein Drink with Strawberries

**INGREDIENTS**

⅓ cup rolled oats

1 scoop of vanilla whey protein

cinnamon powder to taste

1½ cups water

1 stevia packet

4 strawberries, chopped, to decorate

**INSTRUCTIONS**

**1.** In a small pot, add the oats, the whey protein, the cinnamon, and the water. Cook over medium heat for 10 minutes or until thick.

**2.** When the mixture starts to boil, lower the heat and add the stevia and continue to stir with a whisk in order to prevent it from sticking. If it seems too thick, you can give it a whirl in the blender in order to liquefy.

**3.** Accompany with chopped strawberries and enjoy.

YIELD: 1 cup (10½ oz)

| 1,200-CALORIE PLAN | 1,500-CALORIE PLAN | 1,800-CALORIE PLAN |
|---|---|---|
| ▶ ¾ cup (8 oz) | ▶ 1 cup (10½ oz) | ▶ 1¾ cup (18 oz) |

## MEAL 3: LUNCH:
### Buffalo Tenderloin + Sweet Potato Puree + Steamed Green Beans

# buffalo tenderloin

**INGREDIENTS**

16 oz whole buffalo or bison tenderloin

1 tsp garlic, crushed

15 asparagus spears

½ cup mushrooms, chopped

½ cup sun-dried tomatoes, chopped

¼ cup fresh spinach, chopped

1 tbsp pine nuts

1 tbsp BBQ seasoning

pink Himalayan sea salt to taste

pepper to taste

olive oil spray

DAY 1

**INSTRUCTIONS**

**1.** Take the piece of meat and with the help of a sharp knife make a cut down the middle through one of the sides along the length of the piece, as if to create a pocket.

**2.** Fill the "pocket" with the vegetables (garlic, asparagus, mushrooms, tomatoes, spinach, and pine nuts), and season with BBQ powder, salt, and pepper.

**3.** Close the piece with the help of a toothpick, and season on the outside.

**4.** Place the tenderloin on a grill pan sprayed with olive oil over high heat and carefully turn it to sear it on all sides. Then move the meat to the oven and finish cooking.

**5.** Remove the tenderloin from the oven and let it stand for 10 minutes before cutting. It can be accompanied with Sweet Potato Puree and Steamed Green Beans.

**YIELD: 20 oz**

## sweet potato puree

**INGREDIENTS**

15 oz sweet potatoes
4 roasted garlic cloves
¼ cup almond milk
1 pinch of nutmeg
pink Himalayan sea salt to taste
pepper to taste

**INSTRUCTIONS**

**1.** Clean, peel, and wash the sweet potatoes. Cut them into small pieces and steam or microwave them until soft.

**2.** Place the cooked sweet potatoes in a large bowl and add garlic, almond milk, nutmeg, salt, and pepper.

**3.** Use a fork to puree the potatoes or put them in a food processor until you obtain a smooth texture. Serve immediately.

**YIELD: 14.7 oz**

**DAY 1**

# steamed green beans

**INGREDIENTS**

1 cup green beans, cleaned and trimmed
pink Himalayan sea salt to taste
pepper to taste
½ tsp olive oil

**INSTRUCTIONS**

1. Steam the green beans. Add salt, pepper, and olive oil.
2. Serve and enjoy.

YIELD: 7 oz

| 1,200-CALORIE PLAN | 1,500-CALORIE PLAN | 1,800-CALORIE PLAN |
|---|---|---|
| ▶ 4 oz buffalo or bison tenderloin + 2.2 oz sweet potato puree + 5 oz steamed green beans | ▶ 5 oz buffalo or bison tenderloin + 4 oz sweet potato puree + 5 oz steamed green beans | ▶ 6 oz buffalo or bison tenderloin + 6 oz sweet potato puree + 7 oz steamed green beans |

## MEAL 4: SNACK P.M. 1:
### Hard-Boiled Egg Nests with Chicken and Avocado

**INGREDIENTS**

2 hard-boiled eggs, peeled
1 tbsp cooked chicken, shredded
1 tbsp avocado
1 tbsp onion, finely chopped
1 tsp sun-dried tomatoes, finely chopped
juice of ½ lemon
pink Himalayan sea salt to taste
pepper to taste

**INSTRUCTIONS**

1. Take the 2 hard-boiled eggs and cut them in half lengthwise. Discard one yolk and save the other.

2. In a bowl, with the help of a fork, mix the chicken, the reserved yolk, the avocado, the chopped onion, the sun-dried tomatoes, the lemon, the salt, and the pepper until you obtain a homogenous mixture.

3. Place a small scoop of the mixture in each one of the egg halves.

4. Serve and enjoy.

THE HOT BODY DIET

YIELD: 4 egg halves stuffed with chicken and avocado

| 1,200-CALORIE PLAN | 1,500-CALORIE PLAN | 1,800-CALORIE PLAN |
|---|---|---|
| ▶ 2 egg halves | ▶ 3 egg halves | ▶ 4 egg halves |

## MEAL 5: DINNER:
### Zucchini Tortillas + Salmon Tartare

# zucchini tortillas

**INGREDIENTS**

1 cup zucchini
2 whole eggs
6 egg whites
¼ cup almond milk
pink Himalayan sea salt to taste
pepper to taste
1 cup spinach, chopped
1 cup Swiss chard, chopped
olive oil spray

**INSTRUCTIONS**

**1.** Grate the zucchini, and place the pulp in a strainer inside a glass bowl in order to drain the excess liquid. Use a spatula or your hand to apply pressure and drain well.

**2.** In a bowl, with the help of a whisk, beat the eggs and the almond milk, and season with the salt and pepper.

**3.** Add the vegetables to the egg mixture and set aside.

**4.** Heat a nonstick skillet over high heat, spray with olive oil, and add the mixture.

**5.** Lower the heat and allow the tortilla to cook thoroughly, flipping it with a spatula or a plate as needed.

**6.** Place the tortilla on a tray and cut it into triangles.

YIELD: 10 oz

DAY 1

# salmon tartare

## INGREDIENTS

10 oz fresh salmon, skinless, cold or semifrozen
½ cup smoked salmon, chopped
1 tbsp pickles, finely chopped
2 chive sprigs, finely chopped
1 tbsp cilantro, finely chopped
1 sweet pepper, finely chopped
1 hot pepper or jalapeño, finely chopped
juice of 1 lemon
1 tbsp olive oil
1 tsp apple cider vinegar
1 tsp old-fashioned Dijon mustard
1 tsp sriracha sauce
½ tsp lemon zest
chives, chopped, for garnish

## INSTRUCTIONS

**1.** With the help of a good knife, cut the salmon into ¼-inch cubes.

**2.** Place the diced fresh salmon in a bowl and add the chopped smoked salmon, pickles, chives, cilantro, and peppers.

**3.** Prepare the tartare dressing by mixing the lemon juice, the olive oil, the apple cider vinegar, the mustard, the sriracha sauce, and the lemon zest.

**4.** Before serving, whisk together the tartare dressing and add it to the salmon and vegetables. Mix, top with chives, and serve in an ice-cold glass.

YIELD: 14.3 oz

| 1,200-CALORIE PLAN | 1,500-CALORIE PLAN | 1,800-CALORIE PLAN |
|---|---|---|
| ▶ 2½ oz zucchini tortilla + 5.3 oz salmon tartare | ▶ 3½ oz zucchini tortilla + 6.3 oz salmon tartare | ▶ 5 oz zucchini tortilla + 8.4 oz salmon tartare |

## MEAL 6: SNACK P.M. 2:
### Marbled Fit Protein Cupcake

See recipe on page 89.

| 1,200-CALORIE PLAN | 1,500-CALORIE PLAN | 1,800-CALORIE PLAN |
|---|---|---|
| ▶ ½ cupcake | ▶ 1 cupcake | ▶ 1 cupcake* <br> *You can eat a maximum of 1½ cupcakes. |

**DAY 1**

# Day 2

A long journey, a hundred miles long, always starts with a first step. Do it, start today, one day at a time, and you will see that soon you'll become the person you want to be. Just get started and stay on track.

## MEAL 1: PRE-WORKOUT SNACK:
**Egg Whites + Detox Smoothie**

See recipes on page 91.

## MEAL 2: BREAKFAST:
**Spinach Crepe Filled with Turkey and Mushrooms**

**INGREDIENTS**

FOR THE CREPE
⅓ cup rolled oats
¼ cup almond milk
2 egg whites
¼ cup spinach
1 pinch of pink Himalayan sea salt
olive oil spray or coconut oil spray

FOR THE FILLING
6 slices of low-sodium turkey breast ham, cut into small pieces
4 chopped mushrooms
2 tbsp almond mozzarella cheese

**INSTRUCTIONS**

**1.** Place the rolled oats, the almond milk, the egg whites, the spinach, and the salt in a blender and blend for 1 minute.

**2.** Heat a small nonstick skillet over medium heat and add a little olive oil spray or coconut oil spray. Spread a portion of the mixture very thinly across the bottom of the entire pan.

*(Recipe continues)*

DAY 2

**3.** As soon as it starts to brown, use a spatula to flip the crepe and start filling it with the turkey, mushrooms, and almond mozzarella cheese. Fold the crepe in half and cover the pan until the cheese melts.

**4.** Serve and enjoy.

YIELD: 2 crepes with filling (4.8 oz each)

| 1,200-CALORIE PLAN | 1,500-CALORIE PLAN | 1,800-CALORIE PLAN |
|---|---|---|
| ►1½ crepes | ►2 crepes | ►3 crepes |

## MEAL 3: LUNCH:
### Chicken Kebabs + Quinoa Tabbouleh

# chicken kebabs

**INGREDIENTS**

wood skewers
2 tbsps olive oil
1 tbsp garam masala
1 tbsp seven-spice mix (a Middle Eastern mix of paprika, cumin, coriander, cinnamon, cloves, nutmeg, and cardamom)
1 tbsp sumac
1 tbsp of za'atar
1 tbsp crushed garlic
pink Himalayan sea salt to taste
16 oz chicken breast, cubed
1 onion, cut into quarters
1 each red, green, and yellow pepper, diced
olive oil spray

**INSTRUCTIONS**

**1.** Moisten the skewers with water before assembling the kebabs.

**2.** In a large bowl prepare the marinade by mixing the olive oil with the spices (garam masala, seven-spice mix, sumac, and za'atar) as well as the crushed garlic and salt. Set aside.

**3.** Cut the chicken breast into 1-inch cubes. Seal the chicken with the marinade in a bag and let it sit in the refrigerator for at least 4 hours.

**4.** Assemble the skewers in the following order: chicken, onion, red pepper, chicken, green pepper, and so on until you complete the desired pattern.

DAY 2

**5.** Fire up the grill and spray with olive oil, and when it's hot put the skewers on it until they brown on all sides.

**6.** Serve and enjoy.

YIELD: 6 kebabs

# quinoa tabbouleh

### INGREDIENTS

1 cup parsley, finely chopped
1 tbsp chives, finely chopped
1 cup tomatoes, diced
1 cup small cucumber, diced
½ cup cooked quinoa, al dente
1 tbsp lemon juice
1½ tbsps olive oil
pink Himalayan sea salt to taste
pepper to taste

### INSTRUCTIONS

**1.** In a bowl place the parsley and all the fresh vegetables, as well as the quinoa, the lemon juice, the olive oil, and the salt and pepper.

**2.** Mix well and let stand for about 10 minutes.

**3.** When it's time to serve, mix the salad up again to make sure the dressing is properly distributed.

YIELD: 18 oz

| 1,200-CALORIE PLAN | 1,500-CALORIE PLAN | 1,800-CALORIE PLAN |
|---|---|---|
| ▶ 1½ chicken kebabs + 6 oz quinoa tabbouleh | ▶ 2 chicken kebabs + 9 oz quinoa tabbouleh | ▶ 3 chicken kebabs + 12 oz quinoa tabbouleh |

## MEAL 4: SNACK P.M. 1:
### Green Tea Fit Protein Cupcake

See recipe on page 89.

| 1,200-CALORIE PLAN | 1,500-CALORIE PLAN | 1,800-CALORIE PLAN |
|---|---|---|
| ▶ ½ cupcake | ▶ 1 cupcake | ▶ 1 cupcake*<br>*You can eat a maximum of 1½ cupcakes. |

DAY 2

## MEAL 5: DINNER:
### Asian Chicken Cabbage Wraps

**INGREDIENTS**

FOR THE MARINADE

½ cup seedless tamarind paste (sugar-free)

2 stevia packets

2 tbsps rice vinegar

1 tbsp tomato paste

zest and juice of 1 lemon

1 tsp crushed garlic

1 small hot pepper (rocoto, habanero, or jalapeño)

1 tsp natural ginger, grated

FOR THE CHICKEN

24 oz skinless, boneless chicken breast

olive oil spray

1 onion, finely diced

1 red pepper, finely diced

1 garlic clove, diced

¼ cup water

½ cup carrots, grated

½ cup radishes, grated

½ cup red onions, thinly sliced

¼ tbsp apple cider vinegar

pink Himalayan sea salt to taste

zest and juice of 2 lemons

10 large cabbage leaves, washed

¼ cup lentil sprouts

¼ cup unsalted peanuts, chopped (optional)

fresh cilantro to taste

**INSTRUCTIONS**

**1.** Blend all the ingredients for the marinade together. Set aside.

**2.** Cut the chicken breasts into 1-inch cubes and marinate in an airtight bag, in the refrigerator, for 8 to 12 hours. Take the chicken out of the bag and remove any excess marinade.

**3.** Heat a wok with olive oil spray over high heat and toss the chicken until brown. Remove from the heat, set aside, and let cool.

**4.** Cut the chicken into smaller, ¼-inch, cubes until it looks like a hash.

**5.** In the same wok, sauté the onion, the red pepper, and the garlic clove.

**6.** Add the chopped chicken as well as 2 tablespoons of water, then remove from the heat and set aside.

**THE HOT BODY DIET**

DAY 2

**7.** Grab 3 small bowls or cups for the shredded carrots, radishes, and red onion, and put each vegetable in a separate bowl. Add a teaspoon of vinegar, salt, lemon zest, and lemon juice to pickle them slightly. Set aside.

**8.** To assemble the wraps, take a cabbage leaf as if it were a tortilla and add the chicken and the pickled vegetables. Top it off with the sprouts, the chopped peanuts, and the fresh cilantro.

YIELD: 10 cabbage wraps with filling

| 1,200-CALORIE PLAN | 1,500-CALORIE PLAN | 1,800-CALORIE PLAN |
|---|---|---|
| ► 1½ wraps | ► 2 wraps | ► Up to 3 wraps |

## MEAL 6: SNACK P.M. 2:
**Peanut Butter Chocolate Protein Shake**

**INGREDIENTS**

1 cup almond milk or water
1 scoop of chocolate whey protein
1 tsp cocoa powder
1 tsp peanut butter
1–2 stevia packets
½ cup ice, chopped

**INSTRUCTIONS**

**1.** Blend all ingredients for 1 minute.

**2.** Serve and enjoy.

YIELD: 16 oz

| 1,200-CALORIE PLAN | 1,500-CALORIE PLAN | 1,800-CALORIE PLAN |
|---|---|---|
| ► 8 oz | ► 12 oz | ► 16 oz |

DAY 2

## Day 3

A mere wish doesn't change anything; a DECISION changes every-thing. You can spend your entire life wanting to change something, but it isn't until you decide what you want to do and take action that a real change will occur.

## MEAL 1: PRE-WORKOUT SNACK:
**Egg Whites + Detox Smoothie**

See recipes on page 91.

## MEAL 2: BREAKFAST:
**Oatmeal Protein Waffles**

### INGREDIENTS

⅓ cup rolled oats (1.2 oz)
2 egg whites
1 scoop vanilla whey protein
⅓ cup almond milk
½ teaspoon vanilla
1 stevia packet
maple syrup (sugar-free)

### INSTRUCTIONS

**1.** In a blender, blend oatmeal, egg whites, whey protein, almond milk, vanilla, and stevia for 1 minute.

**2.** Heat a waffle pan and spray with vegetable oil. Pour half the mixture into the waffle pan and close. Once the waffle turns golden (or the light on the waffle pan changes from red to green), remove.

**3.** Serve with sugar-free maple syrup and enjoy!

**YIELD: 2 waffles (2.3 oz each)**

| 1,200-CALORIE PLAN | 1,500-CALORIE PLAN | 1,800-CALORIE PLAN |
|---|---|---|
| ► 1 waffle | ► 1½ waffles | ► 2½ waffles |

**Pineapple Shrimp Kebabs + Baked Sweet Potato + Green Salad**

# pineapple shrimp kebabs

### INGREDIENTS

wooden skewers
16 oz shrimp, cleaned and deveined
1 onion, cut in quarters
1 red pepper, cubed
1 green pepper, cubed
1 cup pineapple, chopped
1 yellow pepper, cubed
10 cherry tomatoes
olive oil spray

### INSTRUCTIONS

**1.** Moisten the skewers with water before assembling the kebabs.

**2.** Assemble the skewers in the following order: shrimp, onion, red pepper, another shrimp, green pepper, onion, pineapple, shrimp, and so on until you complete the desired pattern. Top each skewer off with a cherry tomato.

**3.** Fire up the grill, or heat up a frying pan, and spray with olive oil. When it's hot put the skewers on and cook for 2 to 3 minutes on each side. Remove and serve.

**YIELD: 7 kebabs (3.6 oz each)**

# baked sweet potato

### INGREDIENTS

3 large sweet potatoes (5 oz)
olive oil spray
cinnamon
cumin
pink Himalayan sea salt
pepper

*(Recipe continues)*

**DAY 3**

**THE HOT BODY DIET MEAL PLAN**

## INSTRUCTIONS

**1.** Wash and dry the sweet potatoes, keeping the peel on, and cut them in half lengthwise. Spray with olive oil.

**2.** Season with cinnamon, cumin, salt, and pepper to taste.

**3.** Transfer to a baking dish and bake at 350°F for 25 to 30 minutes, until golden brown. (If you have an air fryer, you can use it to bake them for 15 minutes.)

YIELD: 3.3 oz

# green salad

## INGREDIENTS

½ cup tomatoes, chopped
pink Himalayan sea salt to taste
juice and zest of 1 lemon
2 cups mixed greens (lettuce, romaine lettuce, purple cabbage, arugula, watercress, baby spinach, and spinach)
¼ cup alfalfa sprouts
1 tbsp olive oil
1 tbsp apple cider vinegar
pepper to taste

## INSTRUCTIONS

**1.** With the help of a small knife, cut the tomatoes into quarters and add the salt, lemon juice, and lemon zest. Set aside.

**2.** When you're ready to serve, place the tomatoes, mixed greens, and alfalfa sprouts in a large bowl and garnish with olive oil, vinegar, salt, and pepper.

**3.** Serve and enjoy.

YIELD: 2½ cups

| 1,200-CALORIE PLAN | 1,500-CALORIE PLAN | 1,800-CALORIE PLAN |
|---|---|---|
| ▶ 2 pineapple shrimp kebabs + 2.2 oz baked sweet potato + 1 bowl green salad | ▶ 2½ pineapple shrimp kebabs + 4.3 oz baked sweet potato + 1 bowl green salad | ▶ 2 pineapple shrimp kebabs + 6½ oz baked sweet potato + 1 bowl green salad |

DAY 3

THE HOT BODY DIET

## MEAL 4: SNACK P.M. 1:
### Cucumber Wheels + Tuna Avocado Tartare

**INGREDIENTS**

½ large cucumber
1½ oz bluefin tuna, fresh (cold or semifrozen)
1 tsp ginger, grated
½ stalk chives, finely chopped
1 sweet pepper, finely chopped
juice and zest of 1 lemon
½ tsp sesame oil
sriracha sauce
1 tsp soy sauce, low sodium
pepper to taste
1 tbsp avocado, diced
sesame seeds for garnish

**INSTRUCTIONS**

**1.** Wash and cut the cucumber into thick slices. Set aside.

**2.** With the help of a good knife, cut the cold or semifrozen tuna into ¼-inch cubes.

**3.** Transfer to a bowl and add ginger, chives, and sweet pepper.

**4.** Prepare the tartare dressing by mixing the lemon juice, sesame oil, sriracha sauce, lemon zest, soy sauce, and pepper to taste.

**5.** Before serving, beat the tartare dressing thoroughly and add it to the tuna along with the diced avocado. Mix and serve in a chilled glass. Decorate with sesame seeds.

YIELD: 4 cucumber wheels (3 oz) and 3 oz of tartare

| 1,200-CALORIE PLAN | 1,500-CALORIE PLAN | 1,800-CALORIE PLAN |
|---|---|---|
| ▶ 2 cucumber wheels + 1½ oz tuna tartare | ▶ 4 cucumber wheels + 3 oz tuna tartare | ▶ 4 cucumber wheels + 4.6 oz tuna tartare |

DAY 3

# tandoori chicken

**INGREDIENTS**

½ cup nonfat Greek yogurt
1 tbsp garam masala
1 tsp cumin
1 tsp paprika
1 tsp turmeric
1 tsp red pepper flakes
1 tbsp grated ginger
juice and zest of 1 orange
16 oz boneless, skinless chicken breast, cut into 1-inch strips
pink Himalayan sea salt to taste

**INSTRUCTIONS**

**1.** In a large bowl, prepare the marinade by mixing the Greek yogurt with spices, orange juice, and orange zest.

**2.** Put the marinade and the chicken strips in a sealed plastic bag and refrigerate for at least 4 hours.

**3.** Preheat the oven to 350°F. Place the chicken and the marinade in a baking dish, season with salt to taste, and bake in the oven for 30 minutes.

**4.** When the chicken is golden on one side, turn it around until it looks golden on all sides.

**5.** Remove from the oven and serve at the desired degree of doneness.

# greek salad

**FOR THE SALAD**

6 radishes, thinly sliced
½ cup purple onions, thinly sliced
1 garlic clove, crushed
zest of 1 lemon
pink Himalyan sea salt to taste
1 tsp za'atar
1 tbsp apple cider vinegar
1 tsp paprika
2 cups romaine lettuce, chopped
1 bunch of mint

1 cup red, yellow, and orange cherry tomatoes, cut into halves
1 medium cucumber, peeled, seeded, and cut into cubes
¼ cup black olives

FOR THE VINAIGRETTE
⅓ cup apple cider vinegar
1 tbsp extra-virgin olive oil
1 tbsp fresh dill, chopped
pink Himalayan sea salt to taste
pepper to taste

## INSTRUCTIONS

**1.** In a small bowl, place radishes and onions, with a garlic clove, lemon zest, salt, za'atar, 1 tablespoon of vinegar, and paprika. Let stand for 20 to 30 minutes.

**2.** To prepare the vinaigrette, mix the vinegar, olive oil, dill, salt, and pepper in another bowl and set aside.

**4.** In a salad bowl, combine lettuce leaves and mint. Add the radish-and-onion mixture, chopped cherry tomatoes, cucumbers, and olives.

**5.** Mix everything very well.

**6.** Add the vinaigrette before serving, and enjoy.

YIELD: 12 oz of chicken and 5 bowls of salad (1 cup each) with 6 oz

vinaigrette

| 1,200-CALORIE PLAN | 1,500-CALORIE PLAN | 1,800-CALORIE PLAN |
|---|---|---|
| ▶ 4 oz tandoori chicken + 1 bowl Greek salad | ▶ 5 oz tandoori chicken + 1 bowl Greek salad | ▶ 7 oz tandoori chicken + 1 bowl Greek salad |

## MEAL 6: SNACK P.M. 2:
### Chocolate Protein Pancakes

INGREDIENTS
2 egg whites
2 stevia packets
1 scoop of chocolate whey protein
1 tsp unsweetened cocoa powder
olive oil spray

*(Recipe continues)*

DAY 3

**INSTRUCTIONS**

**1.** With the help of an electric mixer at high speed, beat the egg whites until they form soft peaks.

**2.** Decrease the speed and slowly add the stevia, the whey protein, and the cocoa powder.

**3.** Heat a nonstick pan, spray it with olive oil, and add half the mixture. Cover, and when the pancake starts to brown a little, flip it to cook on the other side.

**4.** Serve and enjoy.

**YIELD: 2 pancakes (1.4 oz each)**

**1,200-CALORIE PLAN**
► 1 pancake

**1,500-CALORIE PLAN**
► 2 pancakes

**1,800-CALORIE PLAN**
► 2½ pancakes

# Day 4

The wind can blow away your words, but not even a hurricane can blow away your actions. If you decide you want to do something but don't actually do anything about it, nothing will happen. We'll oftentimes get stuck in our decisions and our wishes and beat ourselves up over our lack of willpower.

## MEAL 1: PRE-WORKOUT SNACK:
**Egg Whites + Detox Smoothie**

See recipes on page 91.

## MEAL 2: BREAKFAST:
**Oatmeal Arepa + Scrambled Eggs**

## oatmeal arepa

**INGREDIENTS**

⅓ cup oat bran
1 egg white
1 scoop vanilla whey protein
1 stevia packet
cinnamon to taste
1 tsp water, for kneading
olive oil spray

**INSTRUCTIONS**

**1.** Mix the oat bran, egg white, whey protein, stevia, cinnamon, and water in a large bowl.

**2.** Knead until you achieve a smooth and dense dough you can use to make small balls that don't stick to your hands. Let stand for 5 minutes.

**3.** Take a piece of dough to make a ball and flatten it between your damp palms in order to shape it into a thin arepa.

**4.** Take a nonstick skillet, spray it with olive oil, and transfer the arepa to cook until golden brown. Flip it and allow it to brown on the other side until it's fully cooked.

DAY 4

# scrambled eggs

**INGREDIENTS**

½ tsp coconut or olive oil
1 egg plus 2 egg whites, beaten
salt to taste
pepper to taste

**INSTRUCTIONS**

**1.** Heat a nonstick skillet with oil, and when the oil is hot, add beaten eggs.

**2.** Gently scramble while adding salt and pepper to taste.

**3.** Serve and enjoy.

YIELD: 1 arepa (3 oz)

| 1,200-CALORIE PLAN | 1,500-CALORIE PLAN | 1,800-CALORIE PLAN |
|---|---|---|
| ▶ 1 egg, 2 egg whites + 1 arepa (3 oz) | ▶ 1 egg, 4 egg whites + 1 arepa (3 oz) | ▶ 1 egg, 6 egg whites + 1 arepa (3 oz) |

## MEAL 3: LUNCH:
### Chicken Quinoa Salad Bowl

**INGREDIENTS**

16 oz chicken breast, diced
1 tsp garlic, crushed
1 tbsp Dijon mustard
1 tsp cilantro, chopped
¼ cup orange juice
olive oil spray
½ cup radicchio, chopped
½ cup endive, finely chopped
½ cup lettuce, chopped
1 grapefruit, peeled and quartered
1 cup quinoa, cooked
alfalfa sprouts to taste
½ cup avocado, diced
basil leaves to taste
apple cider vinegar to taste
pink Himalayan sea salt to taste
pepper to taste

DAY 4

## INSTRUCTIONS

**1.** In a sealed plastic bag, marinate the chicken with the crushed garlic, mustard, cilantro, and orange juice. Refrigerate for at least 4 hours, and then remove the chicken and drain well.

**2.** On a grill or frying pan over high heat, spray with olive oil and sauté the chicken. Stir until all sides are properly cooked and golden. Set aside.

**3.** Place all the vegetables (washed and drained), the quartered grapefruit, cooked quinoa, alfalfa sprouts, avocado, basil leaves, and chicken in a large bowl.

**4.** Season to taste with apple cider vinegar, salt, and freshly ground pepper.

**5.** Serve and enjoy.

YIELD: 13 oz

| 1,200-CALORIE PLAN | 1,500-CALORIE PLAN | 1,800-CALORIE PLAN |
|---|---|---|
| ▶ 9 oz chicken quinoa salad | ▶ 11 oz chicken quinoa salad | ▶ 13 oz chicken quinoa salad |

## MEAL 4: SNACK P.M. 1:
### Strawberry Protein Pancakes

### INGREDIENTS

⅓ cup rolled oats (1.2 oz)
1 whole egg plus 2 egg whites
½ scoop of vanilla whey protein
2 large strawberries, finely chopped
1 tsp chia seeds
½ tsp baking powder
stevia to taste
olive oil spray

### INSTRUCTIONS

**1.** Mix all ingredients except the olive oil spray in a blender.

**2.** Place a nonstick skillet over medium heat and spray it with olive oil. Add a third of the batter.

*(Recipe continues)*

DAY 4

**3.** Cover it, and when the pancake starts to brown a little, flip it immediately to cook the other side.

**4.** Serve and enjoy.

YIELD: 5 pancakes (1.85 oz each)

| 1,200-CALORIE PLAN | 1,500-CALORIE PLAN | 1,800-CALORIE PLAN |
| --- | --- | --- |
| ▶ 1 pancake | ▶ 2 pancakes | ▶ 2½ pancakes |

## MEAL 5: DINNER:
### Grilled Buffalo Ribeye + Pico de Gallo

# grilled buffalo ribeye

**INGREDIENTS**

¼ tsp mustard seeds
¼ tsp peppercorns (black, pink, and green)
1 tsp garlic, crushed
Italian herbs (rosemary, sage, oregano, thyme, and basil) to taste
pink Himalayan sea salt to taste
¼ cup red wine
16 oz buffalo or bison ribeye steak
olive oil spray
½ avocado, chopped, for garnish

**INSTRUCTIONS**

**1.** In a stone mortar or *molcajete*, grind all the spices (mustard seeds, peppercorns, garlic, herbs, and salt) until you obtain a thick paste, and then add the wine. Reserve.

**2.** Place the ribeye steak on a flat surface and rub it with the spice paste, making sure to cover all sides.

**3.** On a grill or in a frying pan sprayed with olive oil, cook the steak over high heat for 5 to 7 minutes on each side until you reach the desired degree of doneness.

**4.** Remove from the heat and let sit for 5 to 8 minutes. Slice and serve along with avocado and Pico de Gallo.

YIELD: 12 oz

# pico de gallo

**INGREDIENTS**

3 tomatoes, diced
½ cup white or purple onion
1 bunch cilantro, finely chopped
2 hot peppers, finely chopped
½ tsp garlic, crushed
juice of 1 lemon
lemon zest to taste
pink Himalayan sea salt to taste
pepper to taste

**INSTRUCTIONS**

**1.** Add the first six ingredients to a bowl and mix.

**2.** Add the lemon zest, salt, and pepper to taste. Transfer to a serving bowl, or to a sealed container if you want to store it in the refrigerator.

YIELD: 1 cup (3½ oz)

| 1,200-CALORIE PLAN | 1,500-CALORIE PLAN | 1,800-CALORIE PLAN |
|---|---|---|
| ► 4 oz buffalo or bison ribeye + 2.3 oz avocado + 1 cup pico de gallo | ► 5 oz buffalo or bison ribeye + 3½ oz avocado + 1 cup pico de gallo | ► 7 oz buffalo or bison ribeye + 4.6 oz avocado + 1 cup pico de gallo |

## MEAL 6: SNACK P.M. 2:

**Peanut Butter Chocolate Protein Balls**

**INGREDIENTS**

¼ cup peanut butter
¼ cup almond flour
1 scoop chocolate whey protein
1 tsp cocoa powder
4 chocolate squares, melted (1.9 oz)
peanuts, chopped, for garnish
nonstick cooking spray

**1.** In a large bowl, combine all ingredients except the cooking spray and stir or use an electric mixer to combine.

**2.** Divide the mixture into eight parts. After coating hands with nonstick cooking spray, roll each portion of the mixture into small balls. If the mixture is very soft, refrigerate for a few minutes before handling.

*(Recipe continues)*

DAY 4

**3.** Once the balls are prepared, they should be stored in an airtight container and refrigerated.

YIELD: 8 balls (0.8 oz each)

1,200-CALORIE PLAN
► 1 protein ball

1,500-CALORIE PLAN
► 1 protein ball

1,800-CALORIE PLAN
► 1½ protein balls

THE HOT BODY DIET

# *Day 5*

It's not about what you should do; it's about what YOU WANT TO DO. You want it because you deserve to live in a light, flexible, strong, and healthy body. It's not about obligations, nor is it about pleasing someone else. To hell with what others might think of you. You're the one who decides what to do with your life.

## MEAL 1: PRE-WORKOUT SNACK:
### Egg Whites + Detox Smoothie

See recipes on page 91.

## MEAL 2: BREAKFAST:
### Chocolate Almond Oatmeal Drink

**INGREDIENTS**

⅓ cup rolled oats (1.2 oz)
1 scoop of chocolate whey protein
1 tsp unsweetened cocoa powder
1½ cups water
2 stevia packets
1 tbsp sliced almonds

**INSTRUCTIONS**

**1.** In a small saucepan, add the rolled oats, whey protein, cocoa powder, and water. Cook over medium heat until thick.

**2.** When it starts to boil, lower the heat, add the stevia, and stir with a whisk or spatula to prevent it from sticking.

**3.** Serve with sliced almonds and enjoy.

**YIELD: 10.7 oz**

| 1,200-CALORIE PLAN | 1,500-CALORIE PLAN | 1,800-CALORIE PLAN |
|---|---|---|
| ▶ 8 oz | ▶ 10.7 oz | ▶ 14½ oz |

# grilled salmon

**INGREDIENTS**

2 salmon fillets, skinless (12 oz)
freshly squeezed juice from 1 orange
1 tbsp ginger, grated
1 garlic clove, grated
1 tsp paprika
zest of 1 orange
olive oil spray
pink Himalayan sea salt to taste
pepper to taste
fresh dill, finely chopped, to taste

**INSTRUCTIONS**

**1.** In a sealed plastic bag, marinate the salmon fillets with the orange juice, ginger, garlic, paprika, and orange zest. Refrigerate for at least 4 hours. Remove the salmon fillets and drain well.

**2.** Next, on the grill or in a frying pan over high heat, spray olive oil and grill the salmon fillets. Season with salt, pepper, and fresh dill.

**3.** Cook the salmon over high heat to sear it on both sides, until it is browned and has reached the desired degree of doneness. Once the salmon is ready, remove from heat, let stand, and serve accompanied with Grilled Asparagus and Sweet Potato Chips.

**YIELD: 16 oz**

# sweet potato chips

**INGREDIENTS**

1 cup sliced sweet potatoes, washed and scrubbed
olive oil spray
pink Himalayan sea salt to taste
pepper to taste
1 tsp oregano

**INSTRUCTIONS**

**1.** With the help of a mandoline or a sharp knife, cut the raw potatoes into thin slices.

DAY 5

**2.** On a perforated tray (such as those used to make pizza) sprayed with olive oil, place the slices and season with salt, pepper, and oregano. Bake at 325°F for 25 minutes or until golden brown, turning from time to time to make sure they don't burn.

**3.** Remove from oven and serve as a side.

YIELD: 7 oz

# grilled asparagus

### INGREDIENTS

20 fresh asparagus spears (16 oz)
2 garlic cloves, crushed
juice of 1 lemon
a pinch of red pepper flakes
pink Himalayan sea salt to taste
olive oil spray

### INSTRUCTIONS

**1.** Wash the asparagus and remove the bottom parts (about an inch).

**2.** Season asparagus with crushed garlic, lemon juice, red pepper flakes, and salt to taste.

**3.** Fire up the grill or heat a nonstick pan over high heat. Spray with olive oil and cook the asparagus for 5 minutes or until crisp.

**4.** Serve and enjoy.

YIELD: 16 oz

| 1,200-CALORIE PLAN | 1,500-CALORIE PLAN | 1,800-CALORIE PLAN |
|---|---|---|
| ▶ 4 oz grilled salmon + 1.7 oz sweet potato chips + 3.3 oz asparagus (7 to 10 spears) | ▶ 5 oz grilled salmon + 3.4 oz sweet potato chips + 5 oz asparagus (10 to 15 spears) | ▶ 7 oz grilled salmon + 5 oz sweet potato chips + 7 oz asparagus (15 to 20 spears) |

## MEAL 4: SNACK P.M. 1:
### Unsalted Nuts

You can choose between unsalted almonds, cashews, pistachios, and peanuts. If you decide to eat only one type of nut, select the portion size according to your calorie plan:

DAY 5

| 1,200-CALORIE PLAN | 1,500-CALORIE PLAN | 1,800-CALORIE PLAN |
|---|---|---|
| ▸Almonds or cashews: 0.8 oz or up to 12 nuts<br>▸Pistachios: ½ oz or up to 25 nuts<br>▸Peanuts (unsalted): ½ oz or up to 20 nuts | ▸Almonds or cashews: 1.3 oz or up to 18 nuts<br>▸Pistachios: 0.8 oz or up to 40 nuts<br>▸Peanuts (unsalted): 0.7 oz or up to 30 nuts | ▸Almonds or cashews: 1.6 oz or up to 24 nuts<br>▸Pistachios: 1 oz or up to 50 nuts<br>▸Peanuts (unsalted): 0.9 oz or up to 40 nuts |

If you want to eat a combination of the four, here are the suggested serving sizes:

| 1,200-CALORIE PLAN | 1,500-CALORIE PLAN | 1,800-CALORIE PLAN |
|---|---|---|
| ▸4 almonds or cashews + 9 pistachios + 6 peanuts (unsalted) | ▸6 almonds or cashews + 14 pistachios + 10 peanuts (unsalted) | ▸8 almonds or cashews + 18 pistachios + 13 peanuts (unsalted) |

## MEAL 5: DINNER:
**Asian Chicken Salad + Asian Vinaigrette**

# asian chicken salad

**INGREDIENTS**

1 cup lettuce, chopped
1 cup kale, chopped
1 cup bok choy, chopped
1 cup daikon radish, julienned
1 cup carrots, julienned
¼ cup radishes, julienned
½ cup purple onions, thinly sliced
½ cup cherry tomatoes, halved
16 oz chicken breast, grilled and sliced
¼ cup soybean sprouts
1 tbsp sesame seeds, toasted
1 tbsp unsalted cashews, chopped
chives, finely chopped, to taste
2 tbsps Asian Vinaigrette (recipe below)

**INSTRUCTIONS**

1. Place all leafy greens and fresh vegetables in a large bowl.

2. Place the sliced grilled chicken fillets on top.

3. Top the salad off by adding the sprouts, the sesame seeds, the cashews, and the chives and season with the vinaigrette (see recipe below).

DAY 5

**THE HOT BODY DIET**

**4.** Mix well and enjoy.

YIELD: 28.6 oz

# asian vinaigrette

**INGREDIENTS**

½ cup rice vinegar
2 tbsps coconut oil
1 tsp lemon grass paste
1 tsp wasabi paste
1 tsp lemon juice
1 tsp ginger paste
2 stevia packets
pink Himalayan sea salt to taste

**INSTRUCTIONS**

In a blender, mix all the ingredients until obtaining a smooth texture. Taste and adjust seasoning, if necessary. Serve or keep in an airtight container in the fridge.

YIELD: 6 oz

| 1,200-CALORIE PLAN | 1,500-CALORIE PLAN | 1,800-CALORIE PLAN |
|---|---|---|
| ▶4.3 oz | ▶5.6 oz | ▶8.6 oz |

## MEAL 6: SNACK P.M. 2:
### Artichoke and Lemon Dip

**INGREDIENTS**

1 artichoke, boiled
juice of 2 lemons
1 tsp olive oil
salt to taste
pepper to taste

**INSTRUCTIONS**

**1.** Boil the artichoke in 1 liter of water for 20 minutes. Remove and drain.

*(Recipe continues)*

DAY 5

**2.** Prepare dressing with lemon juice, olive oil, salt, and pepper.

**3.** Dip the tip of each artichoke leaf in the lemon dressing and enjoy. Once you're done, clean the artichoke heart and eat as well.

**YIELD: 1 artichoke**

**1,200-CALORIE PLAN**
▶ ½ artichoke

**1,500-CALORIE PLAN**
▶ 1 artichoke

**1,800-CALORIE PLAN**
▶ 1½ artichokes

## Day 6

Embark on your journey with joy, not anxiety. You don't have to suffer anymore thinking that you are sacrificing the pleasure of eating. Think of food as high-quality fuel that will make your body work at peak efficiency, and thus help you get rid of excess fat naturally.

## MEAL 1: PRE-WORKOUT SNACK:
**Egg Whites + Detox Smoothie**

See recipes on page 91.

## MEAL 2: BREAKFAST:
**Egg Muffins + High-Fiber Whole Wheat Toast**

### INGREDIENTS

1 egg plus 3 egg whites
¼ cup spinach leaves
2 slices of low-salt turkey breast, thinly sliced (1.55 oz)
0.2 oz sun-dried tomatoes
olive oil spray
0.4 oz vegetarian almond mozzarella cheese
1 slice high-fiber whole wheat toast (½ oz)

### INSTRUCTIONS

**1.** In a bowl, mix the eggs, spinach, thinly sliced turkey breast, and sun-dried tomatoes.

**2.** Spray a silicone muffin tray with a little olive oil spray and pour the egg mixture into the muffin cups.

**3.** Sprinkle the vegetarian cheese on top and bake at 325°F for 20 to 25 minutes or until golden brown.

**4.** Serve with toast and enjoy.

**YIELD: 3 muffins (2.4 oz each)**

| 1,200-CALORIE PLAN | 1,500-CALORIE PLAN | 1,800-CALORIE PLAN |
|---|---|---|
| ▶ 1 muffin + 2 slices of high-fiber whole wheat toast (½ oz each) | ▶ 2 muffins + 3 slices of high-fiber whole wheat toast (½ oz each) | ▶ 2½ muffins + 4 slices of high-fiber whole wheat toast (½ oz each) |

**DAY 6**

# baked chicken thighs

### INGREDIENTS

2 whole chicken thighs, bone-in and with skin (16 oz)
¼ whole rosemary branch
1 tbsp Dijon mustard
juice from 1 lemon
½ head of garlic, cut lengthwise
1 white onion, grated
olive oil spray
1 leek (white parts only)
1 green pepper, julienned
fennel, finely chopped
1 onion, finely chopped
zest of 1 lemon
pink Himalayan sea salt to taste
freshly ground pepper to taste
chicken broth or water to taste (optional)

### INSTRUCTIONS

**1.** In a sealed plastic bag, marinate the chicken thighs with the rosemary, mustard, lemon juice, garlic, and grated onion. Refrigerate for 8 hours.

**2.** Spray a baking dish with olive oil, and then make a bed with the leek, green pepper, fennel, and onion in the dish.

**3.** Place the chicken thighs on top of the vegetable bed. Season with lemon zest, salt, and pepper to taste. Add the juices from the marinade.

**4.** Preheat the oven to 350°F and bake for 45 minutes. If the chicken starts to seem a little dry, you can moisten it with chicken broth or water.

**5.** After 45 minutes, remove the pan from the oven, carefully turn the chicken, and return the dish to the oven for another 15 minutes or until it has reached the desired point of doneness.

YIELD: 13.3 oz

DAY 6

# quinoa

### INGREDIENTS

1 cup quinoa
vegetable oil spray
¼ cup chives, finely chopped
¼ cup hot peppers
1 garlic clove
1½ cup chicken broth
low-sodium salt to taste
pepper to taste

### INSTRUCTIONS

**1.** Wash the quinoa for 2 to 3 minutes or until the water comes out clean. Drain well.

**2.** Heat a nonstick heavy-bottomed pan sprayed with vegetable oil and sauté the chives, hot peppers, and garlic, until slightly brown.

**3.** Add the uncooked quinoa, and toast over high heat for 1 minute, stirring with a wooden spatula.

**4.** Add the chicken broth, the low-sodium salt, and the pepper and wait for the broth to boil and evaporate. Once the broth is absorbed, lower the heat and cover.

**5.** Let it sit for 10 minutes before serving.

**YIELD: 12 oz**

# green salad

See recipe on page 104.

| 1,200-CALORIE PLAN | 1,500-CALORIE PLAN | 1,800-CALORIE PLAN |
|---|---|---|
| ▸4 oz chicken thighs + ½ cup quinoa + 1 bowl green salad | ▸5 oz chicken thighs + 1 cup quinoa + 1 bowl green salad | ▸7 oz chicken thighs + 1½ cups quinoa + 1 bowl green salad |

DAY 6

# MEAL 4: SNACK P.M. 1:
## Chocolate Protein Donut

**INGREDIENTS**

3 egg whites
½ cup stevia
1 egg yolk
1 tsp vanilla
1 tbsp unsweetened cocoa powder
1 scoop chocolate whey protein
1 cup almond flour
1 tsp baking powder
2 tbsps almond milk
2 tbsps chocolate chips (sugar-free)
vegetable oil spray

**INSTRUCTIONS**

**1.** With the help of a hand mixer, beat the egg whites at high speed, until they form soft peaks

**2.** Decrease the speed and slowly add the stevia, egg yolk, vanilla, cocoa, chocolate whey protein, almond flour, baking powder, and almond milk. Beat for 3 minutes.

**3.** Add the chocolate chips and place the mixture in a nonstick donut tray sprayed with vegetable oil.

**4.** Bake at 350°F for 20 to 25 minutes. Allow to cool before serving. Enjoy.

**YIELD: 5 donuts (2.3 oz each)**

| 1,200-CALORIE PLAN | 1,500-CALORIE PLAN | 1,800-CALORIE PLAN |
|---|---|---|
| ►½ donut | ►½ donut | ►1 donut |

# MEAL 5: DINNER:
## Fish Papillote + Julienned Vegetables

### INGREDIENTS

3 golden fish or sea bass fillets (16 oz)

pink Himalayan sea salt to taste

freshly ground black pepper to taste

½ tbsp garlic, crushed

½ tbsp lemongrass paste

½ tbsp ginger, grated

2 cups vegetables (zucchini, peppers, bok choy, celery, chives, garlic, etc.), julienned

1 tsp sriracha sauce

1 tbsp olive oil

zest of 1 lemon

fresh cilantro and/or chives to taste

### INSTRUCTIONS

**1.** Preheat oven to 400°F.

**2.** Season the fish fillets with salt, pepper, garlic, lemongrass, and ginger.

**3.** Season the julienned vegetables with a little salt, and mix well.

**4.** Cut a piece of aluminum foil (approximately 6 inches by 8 inches). Place the fish in the middle of the aluminum foil, season with the sriracha sauce and olive oil, and top off with the vegetables and lemon zest. Do your best to keep about 1 inch free on either side of the aluminum foil.

**5.** Fold the aluminum foil in half and join both ends and sides to create a half-moon shape. Fold over twice, ensuring that the foil is well sealed on all sides.

**6.** Bake for 25 minutes. Remove from the oven and allow to rest for about 5 minutes before opening the papillote. Be very careful when you open it, since the papillote fills up with steam while it's cooking and it can be very hot.

**7.** Serve the fish with the vegetables as well as the cooking liquid. Sprinkle with fresh cilantro and/or chives.

YIELD: 23 oz

| 1,200-CALORIE PLAN | 1,500-CALORIE PLAN | 1,800-CALORIE PLAN |
| --- | --- | --- |
| ▶ 7½ oz | ▶ 8.6 oz | ▶ 13 oz |

DAY 6

# MEAL 6: SNACK P.M. 2:

## Chicken Spinach Burger

### INGREDIENTS

½ cup chicken, cooked and chopped
½ cup raw spinach
¼ red pepper
1 small garlic clove
cilantro to taste
1 tbsp almond flour
1 egg white
salt to taste
pepper to taste
olive oil spray

### INSTRUCTIONS

**1.** Mix all the ingredients except the olive oil spray in a food processor until you obtain a smooth mixture.

**2.** Wash your hands thoroughly, and while they are still damp, form the patties.

**3.** Cook in a nonstick pan sprayed with olive oil. Flip the patties to cook both sides to the desired degree of doneness.

**4.** Serve and enjoy.

**YIELD: 2 burgers (2.35 oz each)**

| 1,200-CALORIE PLAN | 1,500-CALORIE PLAN | 1,800-CALORIE PLAN |
|---|---|---|
| ▶ 1½ burgers | ▶ 2 burgers | ▶ 2½ burgers |

## Day 7

Stop obsessing over achieving the PERFECT BODY and enjoy the achievement of a lean, beautiful, harmonious, strong, and above all healthy body. It's not just about having a beautiful package; the real gift is on the inside. The package is what everyone else sees; the gift is that you are strong and healthy.

## MEAL 1: PRE-WORKOUT SNACK:
### Egg Whites + Detox Smoothie

See recipes on page 91.

## MEAL 2: BREAKFAST:
### Vanilla Cranberry Protein Pancakes

**INGREDIENTS**

⅓ cup rolled oats
1 egg plus 2 egg whites
½ scoop of vanilla whey protein
1 tsp chia seeds
1 tsp flaxseeds
1 tsp stevia
½ tsp vanilla
½ tsp baking powder
1 to 2 tbsps almond milk or water
1 tbsp cranberries
vegetable oil spray

**INSTRUCTIONS**

**1.** Mix all ingredients except the vegetable oil spray in a blender.

**2.** Heat a nonstick skillet over medium heat and spray with vegetable oil. Add a third of the mixture and cover until slightly brown. Immediately flip and cook on the other side.

YIELD: 3 pancakes (2.1 oz each)

| 1,200-CALORIE PLAN | 1,500-CALORIE PLAN | 1,800-CALORIE PLAN |
|---|---|---|
| ▶ 1½ pancakes | ▶ 2 pancakes | ▶ 3 pancakes |

DAY 7

# MEAL 3: LUNCH:
## Red Tuna, Wakame, Quinoa Salad

### INGREDIENTS

¼ cup lemon juice

¼ cup orange juice

1 tbsp light soy sauce

1 tsp sesame oil

1 tbsp wasabi paste

1 tbsp sriracha sauce

1 tbsp rice vinegar or mirin

1 tsp ginger, grated

zest of 1 lemon

16 oz redfin tuna, cubed (very cold, semifrozen)

½ cup red pepper, finely chopped

½ cup yellow pepper, finely chopped

½ cup cucumber, peeled and seeded, finely chopped

¼ cup celery, finely chopped

¼ cup onion, finely chopped

¼ cup chives, finely chopped

1 tbsp cilantro, finely chopped

1 cup Quinoa (see recipe on page 123)

½ cup wakame

1 tbsp sesame seeds

### INSTRUCTIONS

**1.** In a bowl, prepare the dressing by whisking together the lemon juice, orange juice, soy sauce, sesame oil, wasabi, sriracha sauce, rice vinegar, ginger, and lemon zest. Keep refrigerated.

**2.** With the help of a good knife, cut the very cold, semifrozen tuna into cubes.

**3.** In a stainless steel bowl, combine the tuna cubes and the dressing. Set aside and keep refrigerated for at least 10 minutes.

**4.** In another bowl, mix the peppers, cucumber, celery, onion, chives, cilantro, and Quinoa.

**5.** Top the salad with the tuna, wakame, and sesame seeds.

YIELD: 4 salad bowls (10.8 oz each)

| 1,200-CALORIE PLAN | 1,500-CALORIE PLAN | 1,800-CALORIE PLAN |
|---|---|---|
| ▶ 1 bowl (10.8 oz) | ▶ 1½ bowls (16 oz) | ▶ 2 bowls (22 oz) |

DAY 7

## MEAL 4: SNACK P.M. 1:

**Popcorn**

### INGREDIENTS

5 tbsps popcorn kernels
5 tbsps water
salt to taste
pepper to taste

### INSTRUCTIONS

**1.** Place the popcorn kernels in a large, round, microwave-safe container.

**2.** Add the water, the salt, and the pepper to taste.

**4.** Cover the container with plastic film, making sure it's perfectly sealed around the edges. Then with a sharp knife pierce the film 4 or 5 times.

**5.** Microwave for 5 minutes. Remove the plastic film, serve, and enjoy! The container gets very hot, so be careful when you remove it from the microwave!

YIELD: 3 cups (1.8 oz each)

| 1,200-CALORIE PLAN | 1,500-CALORIE PLAN | 1,800-CALORIE PLAN |
|---|---|---|
| ►1 cup | ►2 cups | ►3 cups |

## MEAL 5: DINNER:

**Turkey Stew + Mixed Salad**

# turkey stew

See recipe on page 131.

# mixed salad

**INGREDIENTS**

½ cup Roma tomatoes, chopped
pink Himalayan sea salt to taste
juice and zest of 1 lemon
2 cups mixed greens (romaine lettuce, purple cabbage, watercress, baby spinach, and endive)
¼ cup alfalfa sprouts
1 tbsp olive oil
1 tbsp apple cider vinegar
fresh pepper to taste

**INSTRUCTIONS**

**1.** Use a small knife to quarter the tomatoes. Add salt, lemon zest, and lemon juice. Set aside.

**2.** When you are ready to serve, place the mixed greens, the tomatoes, and the alfalfa sprouts in a large bowl. Dress with olive oil, vinegar, salt, and pepper.

YIELD: 2½ bowls of salad (6 oz each)

| 1,200-CALORIE PLAN | 1,500-CALORIE PLAN | 1,800-CALORIE PLAN |
|---|---|---|
| ▶ 4.2 oz turkey stew + 1 bowl mixed salad | ▶ 5.6 oz turkey stew + 1 bowl mixed salad | ▶ 7.2 oz turkey stew + 1 bowl mixed salad |

## MEAL 6: SNACK P.M. 2:
### Turkey Asparagus Rolls

**INGREDIENTS**

2 slices turkey breast ham
2 black Kalamata olives, chopped
2 sun-dried tomatoes, chopped
2 asparagus spears, cooked
alfalfa sprouts to taste
1 tsp mustard

**INSTRUCTIONS**

**1.** Lay out the 2 slices of turkey ham and add 1 olive, 1 sun-dried tomato, 1 asparagus spear, and a pinch of alfalfa sprouts.

**2.** Roll up carefully and serve with mustard to taste.

YIELD: 2 rolls (1.3 oz each)

| 1,200-CALORIE PLAN | 1,500-CALORIE PLAN | 1,800-CALORIE PLAN |
|---|---|---|
| ▶ 2½ rolls | ▶ 3½ rolls | ▶ 4½ rolls |

**DAY 7**

## SUPERSTAR RECIPE OF THE WEEK

# chicken, turkey, or tuna stew

### INGREDIENTS

olive oil spray
Italian spices: oregano, red pepper flakes, basil, sage, rosemary
1 cup onions, finely chopped
1 cup leeks, finely chopped
1 cup sweet peppers, chopped
½ cup chives, finely chopped
1 cup red pepper, finely chopped
1 cup celery, finely chopped
4 garlic cloves, minced
1 large tomato, finely chopped
pink Himalayan sea salt to taste
pepper to taste
3 cups cooked chicken breast, ground turkey, or well-drained tuna
1 tbsp mustard
1 tbsp tomato paste
1 tbsp balsamic vinegar
1 cup chicken or vegetable broth
cilantro, finely chopped, to taste

### INSTRUCTIONS

**1.** Heat a nonstick skillet or thick-bottomed pan sprayed with olive oil over medium heat. Add the Italian spices and sauté for 1 minute.

**2.** Add the onions, leeks, sweet peppers, chives, red pepper, celery, garlic, and tomato. Add pink Himalayan sea salt and pepper to taste.

**3.** Incorporate the tuna, turkey, or chicken breast, along with the mustard, tomato paste, and balsamic vinegar.

**4.** Add the broth and allow it to reduce. Adjust the seasoning and add the finely chopped cilantro to taste.

YIELD: 26 oz turkey stew • 24 oz chicken stew • 19 oz tuna stew

## Day 8

You are your own star. Don't expect to be perfect; nobody is. Don't try to imitate anyone, not even me. Simply strive to do your best regardless of the task at hand. Did it go right? Thank yourself. Did it go wrong? Try again, but don't feel frustrated. If something doesn't turn out as you expected, don't worry. Just start again, as many times as necessary!

### MEAL 1: PRE-WORKOUT SNACK:
**Egg Whites + Apple Green Tea Infusion**

See Egg Whites recipe on page 91.

## apple green tea infusion

**INGREDIENTS**

2 green apples, seeded and peeled
4 cups of water
4 cinnamon sticks
½ cup hibiscus flowers
2 tbsps matcha tea or 8 green tea bags
lemon to taste
stevia to taste

**INSTRUCTIONS**

**1.** Cut the apples into quarters.

**2.** Place the quartered apples, water, and cinnamon sticks in a saucepan over high heat and bring to a boil.

**3.** Once the water is boiling, remove the saucepan from the heat and add the hibiscus flowers and tea.

**4.** Allow the tea to cool and add lemon and/or stevia to taste.

**5.** Serve and enjoy.

YIELD: 34 oz

| 1,200-CALORIE PLAN | 1,500-CALORIE PLAN | 1,800-CALORIE PLAN |
|---|---|---|
| ▸8 oz | ▸12 oz | ▸16 oz |

DAY 8

# MEAL 2: BREAKFAST:

## Quinoa Arepa + Tomato Scrambled Eggs

### INGREDIENTS

1 cup cooked quinoa

½ cup oat bran or cornmeal

1 egg white

1 tbsp chia seeds

1 tbsp flaxseeds

1 tbsp hemp seeds

⅓ cup water, for kneading

olive oil spray

2 tbsps chives or leeks, chopped

2 tbsps tomatoes, chopped

3 egg whites plus 1 yolk

pink Himalayan sea salt to taste

pepper to taste

### INSTRUCTIONS

**1.** Cook the quinoa following the directions on the package. Reserve 1 cup of cooked quinoa for this recipe.

**2.** In a bowl or processor, mix the quinoa with oat bran or cornmeal, 1 egg white, chia seeds, flaxseeds, hemp seeds, and water. Mix well until you obtain a smooth dough you can use to make arepas.

**3.** Take a piece of dough to make a ball and flatten it between your damp palms in order to shape it into a thin arepa.

**4.** Take a nonstick skillet, spray it with olive oil, and transfer the arepa to cook until golden brown. Flip it and allow it to brown on the other side until it's fully cooked.

**5.** In another nonstick skillet sprayed with olive oil, add the chives and tomatoes and cook for 1 minute. Then add the remaining eggs, salt, and pepper to taste. Mix with a spatula until thoroughly cooked.

**6.** Serve with the arepas and enjoy.

YIELD: Arepas: 3 arepas (4.15 oz each) and 6.7 oz eggs

| 1,200-CALORIE PLAN | 1,500-CALORIE PLAN | 1,800-CALORIE PLAN |
|---|---|---|
| ▶ 1 quinoa arepa + 6 oz scrambled eggs | ▶ 2 quinoa arepas + 9 oz scrambled eggs | ▶ 3 quinoa arepas + 12 oz scrambled eggs |

DAY 8

# chicken chili

**INGREDIENTS**

olive oil spray
1 tbsp chili powder, spicy
1 tsp chili seasoning
1 tsp ground chipotle
1 tbsp powdered paprika
1 tsp ground cumin
2½ cups ground chicken breast
pink Himalayan sea salt to taste
pepper to taste
½ cup onion, diced
½ cup leeks, finely diced
½ cup sweet chilies, diced
½ cup chives, finely chopped
¼ cup red paprika, diced
½ cup celery, diced
2 garlic cloves, minced
2 cups tomatoes, crushed
1 cup fresh red pepper pulp, grated
½ tbsp mustard
¼ cup tomato paste
½ tbsp balsamic vinegar
4 cups water or chicken, beef, or vegetable broth
fresh chives, finely chopped, to taste
cilantro, finely chopped, to taste

**INSTRUCTIONS**

**1.** Heat a nonstick skillet or large heavy-bottomed pan over medium heat and spray with olive oil. Stir the powdered spices first (chili powder, chili seasoning, chipotle, paprika, and cumin), without letting them burn.

**2.** Add the ground chicken, using a spatula or wooden spoon to break it apart. Cook and brown it completely.

**3.** Add salt and pepper to taste. Remove and set aside.

**4.** Spray some olive oil onto the same pan and add onion, leeks, sweet chilies, chives, red paprika, celery, garlic, tomatoes, and red pepper pulp and cook over medium heat for 10 minutes or until it looks creamy.

**DAY 8**

**5.** Add the chicken, mustard, tomato paste, and balsamic vinegar.

**6.** Lower the heat completely and add the water or broth. Cook for at least an hour, making sure it doesn't stick to the pan. Allow the broth to reduce, adjust the seasoning, and add the finely chopped chives and cilantro to taste.

YIELD: 40 oz

# stuffed baked potatoes

### INGREDIENTS

2 medium potatoes (10½ oz)
olive oil spray
pink Himalayan sea salt to taste
dried or fresh herbs (oregano, thyme, rosemary, sage) to taste
1 tbsp nonfat Greek yogurt (optional)

### INSTRUCTIONS

**1.** Thoroughly wash and scrub the potatoes. With a knife mark a cross or X on the top of each.

**2.** Spray with the olive oil and season with salt and herbs to taste. Wrap each potato individually in aluminum foil.

**3.** Bake at 350°F for 35 to 45 minutes until you reach the desired doneness. You can pierce with a knife to check.

**4.** Remove the potatoes from the oven and, using a knife and being careful not to burn yourself, cut an X across the top of each and peel away the aluminum foil. Make room to stuff the potato with the Chicken Chili, and top with the cilantro and fresh chives. If you wish to do so, you can add 1 tablespoon of nonfat Greek yogurt.

**5.** Serve and enjoy.

YIELD: 2 potatoes (5 oz each)

# green salad

See recipe on page 104.

| 1,200-CALORIE PLAN | 1,500-CALORIE PLAN | 1,800-CALORIE PLAN |
|---|---|---|
| ▶ ½ medium (6 oz) potato filled with 5 oz chicken chili + 1 bowl green salad | ▶ 1 medium (6 oz) potato filled with 6.3 oz chicken chili + 1 bowl green salad | ▶ 1½ medium (6 oz) potatoes filled with 9 oz chicken chili + 1 bowl green salad |

DAY 8

## MEAL 4: SNACK P.M. 1:
### Pineapple Fit Protein Cupcake

See recipe on page 89.

| 1,200-CALORIE PLAN | 1,500-CALORIE PLAN | 1,800-CALORIE PLAN |
|---|---|---|
| ▶ ½ cupcake | ▶ 1 cupcake | ▶ 1 cupcake*<br>*You can eat a maximum of 1½ cupcakes |

## MEAL 5: DINNER:
### Chicken-Stuffed Portobello Mushrooms + Pico de Gallo

**INGREDIENTS**

4 large portobello mushrooms
olive oil spray
1 cup Chicken Stew (see recipe on page 131)
1 tbsp Pico de Gallo (see recipe on page 113)

**INSTRUCTIONS**

**1.** Wash and wipe the portobellos with a damp cloth. Remove the stems and use a teaspoon to remove the brown gills from the insides of the mushrooms.

**2.** Fire up the grill or heat a nonstick skillet over high heat. Spray the portobellos with olive oil and quickly sear them on both sides. Remove and set aside.

**3.** After grilling the portobellos, place them with the stem sides up in order to fill each one with ¼ cup Chicken Stew and top with the Pico de Gallo.

**YIELD: 4 stuffed portobellos (3.6 oz each)**

| 1,200-CALORIE PLAN | 1,500-CALORIE PLAN | 1,800-CALORIE PLAN |
|---|---|---|
| ▶ 2 stuffed portobello mushrooms (3.6 oz each) + ½ cup pico de gallo | ▶ Up to 3 stuffed portobello mushrooms (3.6 oz each) + 1 cup pico de gallo | ▶ Up to 4 stuffed portobello mushrooms (3.6 oz each) + 1 cup pico de gallo |

DAY 8

## MEAL 6: SNACK P.M. 2:
### Lettuce Turkey Rolls

**INGREDIENTS**

4 leaves of romaine lettuce
4 oz Turkey Stew (see recipe on page 131)
½ cup arugula
5 cherry tomatoes cut into halves
mustard to taste
za'atar to taste

**INSTRUCTIONS**

1. Take a lettuce leaf and fill it with Turkey Stew.

2. Top with arugula, cherry tomatoes, mustard, and za'atar.

3. Serve and enjoy.

YIELD: 4 stuffed lettuce leaves (1.45 oz each)

| 1,200-CALORIE PLAN | 1,500-CALORIE PLAN | 1,800-CALORIE PLAN |
|---|---|---|
| ▶ Up to 2 lettuce turkey rolls | ▶ Up to 4 lettuce turkey rolls | ▶ Up to 6 lettuce turkey rolls |

DAY 8

## Day 9

Think about how you're going to look in those jeans that haven't fit you in a while. Find a garment that doesn't fit, or buy a pair of jeans that is a size smaller than your current size. Leave it in a visible place and try it on every week, until the day comes when you are able to fit into it. That day you will feel more powerful than ever.

## MEAL 1: PRE-WORKOUT SNACK:
### Egg Whites + Apple Green Tea Infusion

See Egg Whites recipe on page 91 and Apple Green Tea Infusion recipe on page 132.

## MEAL 2: BREAKFAST:
### Tuna Yucca Fritters

**INGREDIENTS**

1 cup cooked yucca, mashed
1 egg white
½ cup cornmeal or oat bran
1 tbsp chia seeds
1 tbsp flaxseeds
1 tbsp hemp seeds
pink Himalayan sea salt to taste
pepper to taste
2–3 tbsps water, for kneading
½ cup Tuna Stew (4¼ oz) (see recipe on page 131)
olive oil spray

**INSTRUCTIONS**

**1.** In a bowl or with the help of a food processor, mix the mashed yucca with the egg white, cornmeal or oat bran, chia seeds, flaxseeds, hemp seeds, salt, pepper, and water. If the dough becomes too tough, add more water.

**2.** Knead well until the dough feels smooth like clay.

**3.** With wet hands, take a portion of the dough and shape it into a ball. Then open a wide hole in the middle with your fingers, and fill with a spoonful of Tuna Stew. Close the hole back up until you have a perfectly round ball again.

DAY 9

**4.** Heat a frying pan and spray it with olive oil. Fry the fritters until they are brown on all sides. Then put them in the oven at 350°F for 25 minutes to finish cooking. If you have an air fryer, you can use it for this last stage instead of the oven.

**5.** Serve and enjoy.

YIELD: 6 fritters (1.65 oz each) + ½ cup tuna stew (4¼ oz)

| 1,200-CALORIE PLAN | 1,500-CALORIE PLAN | 1,800-CALORIE PLAN |
|---|---|---|
| ▶ 2 fritters | ▶ 3½ fritters | ▶ 5 fritters |

## MEAL 3: LUNCH:
**Buffalo Fajitas + Brown Rice + Steamed Broccoli**

# buffalo fajitas

### INGREDIENTS
olive oil spray
½ tsp powdered paprika
½ tsp BBQ seasoning
16 oz buffalo or bison steak, clean and cut into thin slices
½ cup onion, julienned
½ cup red pepper, julienned
½ cup green pepper, julienned
1 tsp sriracha sauce
a pinch of pink Himalayan sea salt (optional)
¼ cup water, to deglaze (optional)
fresh parsley, finely chopped, for garnish

### INSTRUCTIONS

**1.** Heat a skillet or griddle over high heat and spray it with olive oil.

**2.** Add paprika and BBQ seasoning. Next, add the buffalo steak to the pan in batches, in order to make sure everything grills properly. Remove from the heat and set aside.

**3.** Sauté the onions and peppers in the same skillet until the vegetables are brown or transparent, at which point you can transfer the sliced steak to the mix.

*(Recipe continues)*

**DAY 9**

**4.** Finish by seasoning with the sriracha. If you want, add a pinch of salt and the water to deglaze the juices from the cooking surface. Add finely chopped fresh parsley.

**5.** Serve and enjoy.

YIELD: 23 oz

# brown rice

### INGREDIENTS

olive oil spray
½ onion, finely diced
1 garlic clove, crushed
2 sweet peppers, finely chopped
1 cup uncooked brown rice (washed and well drained)
2½ cups broth or water
pink Himalayan sea salt to taste

### INSTRUCTIONS

**1.** In a medium saucepan, spray olive oil and sauté the onion, the garlic clove, and the sweet peppers over medium heat.

**2.** Add the brown rice. Sauté for 1 minute. Then add the 2½ cups of broth or water. Season with salt, to taste.

**3.** Let the mixture boil uncovered, until the broth is absorbed. Then cover, lower the heat to a minimum, and cook for 10 to 15 minutes more.

**4.** Serve immediately and enjoy.

YIELD: 14 oz cooked rice

# steamed broccoli

### INGREDIENTS

2 cups of broccoli
pinch of pink Himalayan sea salt
1 tbsp olive oil
pepper to taste

### INSTRUCTIONS

**1.** Cut the broccoli into florets.

**2.** Fill a large pot with two inches of water and a pinch of salt and bring to a boil.

**3.** Once the water boils, add the broccoli and cover. Allow to boil for five minutes.

**4.** Turn off the heat and drain the broccoli in a colander. Top with olive oil and pepper. Serve and enjoy.

YIELD: 2 cups of broccoli

| 1,200-CALORIE PLAN | 1,500-CALORIE PLAN | 1,800-CALORIE PLAN |
|---|---|---|
| ▶ 5½ oz buffalo fajitas + 2 oz brown rice + steamed broccoli | ▶ 6½ oz buffalo fajitas + 4 oz brown rice + steamed broccoli | ▶ 8½ oz buffalo fajitas + 6 oz brown rice + steamed broccoli |

## MEAL 4: SNACK P.M. 1:
### Tzatziki + Carrot Sticks

**INGREDIENTS**

½ cucumber, skinless, seedless
½ cup nonfat Greek yogurt
1 tsp olive oil
juice of 1 lemon
1 small garlic clove, crushed
¼ tsp za'atar
pink Himalayan sea salt to taste
1¼ cups finely chopped dill and/or peppermint leaves
pepper to taste
carrot, cut into sticks

**INSTRUCTIONS**

**1.** Grate the cucumber, place it in a strainer, and let it drain. Discard the water.

**2.** Place cucumbers, yogurt, olive oil, lemon juice, garlic, and za'atar in a bowl; mix with a spoon, and add salt to taste.

**3.** When you are ready to serve, sprinkle with the dill and/or peppermint and black pepper.

**4.** Dip the carrots in the tzatziki and enjoy.

YIELD: 7.3 oz

| 1,200-CALORIE PLAN | 1,500-CALORIE PLAN | 1,800-CALORIE PLAN |
|---|---|---|
| ▶ Up to 5 oz tzatziki | ▶ Up to 7½ oz tzatziki | ▶ Up to 10 oz tzatziki |

DAY 9

## MEAL 5: DINNER:

**Chicken Chili–Stuffed Tomatoes + Vegetarian Cheese**

### INGREDIENTS

6 large tomatoes
1½ cups spinach, chopped
1½ cups Chicken Chili (see recipe on page 134)
1 cup almond cheese, grated (vegetarian cheese)
olive oil spray

### INSTRUCTIONS

**1.** With the help of a sharp knife, cut off the tops of the tomatoes. Use a spoon to remove the seeds and the pulp, leaving them ready to be stuffed.

**2.** Place a bed of chopped spinach (¼ cup) in each tomato. Then fill it with the Chicken Chili (¼ cup) and top with the grated vegetarian cheese.

**3.** Preheat the oven to broil. Spray a nonstick pan or baking dish with olive oil, place the stuffed tomatoes in it, and put it in the oven for broiling.

**4.** Once the cheese starts to brown, remove and serve.

YIELD: 6 stuffed tomatoes (5 oz each)

| 1,200-CALORIE PLAN | 1,500-CALORIE PLAN | 1,800-CALORIE PLAN |
|---|---|---|
| ▶ 1 stuffed tomato | ▶ 1½ stuffed tomatoes | ▶ 2 stuffed tomatoes |

## MEAL 6: SNACK P.M. 2:

**Light Blackberry Gelatin**

### INGREDIENTS

2 cups water
1 box of your favorite flavor gelatin, sugar-free
½ cup whole fresh blackberries

### INSTRUCTIONS

**1.** Heat 1 cup of water.

**2.** In a large bowl, mix 1 cup of hot water with 1 cup of cold water and then add the gelatin box and the fresh blackberries.

**3.** Refrigerate until cool and firm. Serve and enjoy.

YIELD: 4 cups (8 oz each)

| 1,200-CALORIE PLAN | 1,500-CALORIE PLAN | 1,800-CALORIE PLAN |
|---|---|---|
| ▶ Up to 2 cups | ▶ Up to 4 cups | ▶ Up to 6 cups |

DAY 9

## Day 10

Dreams don't just come true. You have to WORK FOR THEM. Only rain and snow fall from the sky. You must work with passion and persistence to achieve what you want, and the result will depend on the effort you put into it. Think about it: how much am I willing to put in?

## MEAL 1: PRE-WORKOUT SNACK:
### Egg Whites + Apple Green Tea Infusion

See Egg Whites recipe on page 91 and Apple Green Tea Infusion recipe on page 132.

## MEAL 2: BREAKFAST:
### Green Plantain Turkey Empanadas

**INGREDIENTS**

1 cup cooked green plantain, mashed
1 egg white
½ cup cornmeal or oat bran
1 tbsp chia seeds
1 tbsp flaxseeds
1 tbsp hemp seeds
2–3 tbsps water, for kneading
pink Himalayan sea salt to taste
pepper to taste
⅓ cup water
½ cup Turkey Stew (see recipe on page 131)
olive oil spray

**INSTRUCTIONS**

**1.** In a bowl or with the help of a food processor, mix the mashed plantain with the egg white, cornmeal or oat bran, chia seeds, flaxseeds, hemp seeds, salt, pepper, and water. If the dough becomes too tough, add more water.

**2.** Knead well until the dough feels smooth like clay.

**3.** Shape the patties with wet hands, taking portions of the dough and making balls. Flatten onto a plastic bag (cut it in two with scissors so you have two pieces) previously sprayed with olive oil.

**4.** Place the second piece of the plastic bag on top of the flattened dough and pass a rolling pin over it until you have a large disk that's about ¼ inch thick.

**5.** Remove the disk from between the pieces of plastic and place it on an empanada press (available at any cooking store). In the center add 1 tablespoon of Turkey Stew and close the press, squeezing it well.

**6.** Carefully remove the empanada from the press, spray it with olive oil, and bake it at 350°F for 25 minutes. If you have an air fryer and you'd like to use it instead of the oven, cook the empanada in the air fryer until it's golden brown and crispy.

**7.** Serve and enjoy.

**YIELD: 3 empanadas (5.3 oz each)**

| 1,200-CALORIE PLAN | 1,500-CALORIE PLAN | 1,800-CALORIE PLAN |
| --- | --- | --- |
| ▶ 1 empanada | ▶ 1½ empanadas | ▶ 2 empanadas |

## MEAL 3: LUNCH:
**Crispy Fish Sticks + Baked Yucca Fries + Pico de Gallo**

# crispy fish sticks

### INGREDIENTS

3 whitefish fillets (dorado, corvina, sea bass, or tilapia) (16 oz)
pink Himalayan sea salt to taste
pepper to taste
1 cup dry coconut, coarsely grated
1 oz high-fiber whole wheat bread crumbs
¼ cup mustard, coriander, pepper seeds, and ground peperoncino
zest of 1 lemon
1 egg plus 2 egg whites, beaten
olive oil spray

### INSTRUCTIONS

**1.** Cut the fish into sticks (approximately ⅓ inch x 1 inch). Season with salt and pepper and set aside in the refrigerator.

**2.** In a large bowl, mix the coconut, bread crumbs, the spice mix, and lemon zest.

*(Recipe continues)*

DAY 10

**3.** Bread the fish sticks: dip them in the egg mixture and then the grated coconut mix in order to form a coconut crust; make sure that it covers all sides of each fish stick. Place the fish sticks on a tray and set aside.

**4.** Preheat the oven to 350°F. Spray the bottom of a nonstick baking dish with olive oil and place the breaded fish sticks inside. Bake them in the oven until golden brown on all sides.

**5.** Serve and enjoy.

YIELD: 4 servings (4 oz each)

## baked yucca fries

### INGREDIENTS

7 oz yucca, peeled and clean
1 bunch of fresh parsley, chopped
pink Himalayan sea salt to taste
pepper to taste
olive oil spray

### INSTRUCTIONS

**1.** Use a sharp knife to cut yucca into thin fry shapes.

**2.** Place the yucca fries in a nonstick baking dish, season with parsley, salt, and pepper, and spray with olive oil.

**3.** Broil the yucca fries in the oven for 8 to 10 minutes, turning them from time to time and making sure they don't burn. Once they turn golden brown on all sides, take them out of the oven and serve as a side. (You can also fry them in an air fryer if you have one.)

**4.** Serve and enjoy.

YIELD: 3.8 oz

## pico de gallo

See recipe on page 113.

| 1,200-CALORIE PLAN | 1,500-CALORIE PLAN | 1,800-CALORIE PLAN |
|---|---|---|
| ▶ 3½ oz crispy fish sticks + 1.3 oz baked yucca fries + ½ cup pico de gallo | ▶ 4.2 oz crispy fish sticks + 2.6 oz baked yucca fries + 1 cup pico de gallo | ▶ 6 oz crispy fish sticks + 4 oz baked yucca fries + 1 cup pico de gallo |

DAY 10

## MEAL 4: SNACK P.M. 1:
### Peanut Butter Blondies

**INGREDIENTS**

¼ cup peanut butter
¼ cup stevia
2 tbsps unsweetened syrup
2 eggs
1 tbsp vanilla extract
2 cups almond flour
2 tbsps almond milk
½ tsp salt
½ tsp baking powder

**INSTRUCTIONS**

**1.** Using an electric mixer, mix peanut butter, stevia, unsweetened syrup, eggs, and vanilla extract. Beat for 2 minutes.

**2.** Add the almond flour, almond milk, salt, and baking powder. Continue beating for another minute.

**3.** Transfer to a baking dish and bake at 325°F for 25 minutes until lightly brown. Let cool, cut, and serve.

**YIELD: 12 blondies (1.15 oz each)**

| 1,200-CALORIE PLAN | 1,500-CALORIE PLAN | 1,800-CALORIE PLAN |
|---|---|---|
| ►1 blondie | ►1 blondie | ►1½ blondies |

## MEAL 5: DINNER:
### Turkey Meatballs with Tomato Ragout + Zucchini Noodles

# zucchini noodles

**INGREDIENTS**

3 zucchini

**INSTRUCTIONS**

Wash the zucchini without peeling them, and with the help of a spiralizer turn them into noodles. A spiralizer is a kitchen gadget that helps make vegetable noodles, but if you don't have one you can make them by cutting the zucchini into long, thin slices with a sharp knife.

DAY 10

# turkey meatballs

**INGREDIENTS**

1 cup white onion, diced
¼ cup chives
¼ cup celery, chopped
¼ cup garlic, finely chopped
½ cup sweet peppers, finely chopped
1 tbsp water
16 oz ground turkey
pink Himalayan sea salt to taste
pepper to taste
olive oil spray

**INSTRUCTIONS**

**1.** In a blender, process the onion, chives, celery, garlic, sweet peppers, and water until you have a smooth consistency.

**2.** In a large bowl, add half the ground turkey meat and ¼ cup of the vegetable blend. Mix with your hands and season with salt and pepper.

**3.** Shape the meatballs by taking small portions of prepared turkey and forming them into small balls with the palms of your wet hands (this should prevent sticking).

**4.** In a large nonstick skillet sprayed with olive oil, cook the meatballs until they turn golden brown. Remove from heat and reserve. Repeat with the remaining ingredients.

# tomato ragout

**INGREDIENTS**

olive oil spray
Italian spices (oregano, sage, thyme, rosemary, and red pepper flakes) to taste
½ cup red pepper, chopped
4 garlic cloves, roasted
4 cups tomatoes, peeled and seeded
8 fresh basil leaves
1 tbsp balsamic vinegar
2 tbsps tomato paste
1 bay leaf
1 stevia packet
1 tsp Dijon mustard
pink Himalayan sea salt to taste
pepper to taste
fresh basil, finely chopped, to taste

**INSTRUCTIONS**

**1.** Spray the same skillet you used to make the meatballs with olive oil and add the Italian spices.

**2.** Add the red pepper, roasted garlic cloves, tomatoes, and fresh basil and cook over medium heat for 5 minutes. Then put in a blender and blend for 1 minute.

**3.** Transfer the meatballs and the sauce, from the blender, back to the skillet. Cook uncovered, over low heat, for 30 minutes or until the ragout evaporates a little.

**4.** Add the balsamic vinegar, tomato paste, bay leaf, stevia, and mustard to the ragout while it's cooking. Reduce until it attains the desired consistency. Season with salt and pepper and remove from heat.

**5.** In a bowl or deep dish, serve the zucchini noodles with the ragout and meatballs on top. Sprinkle with the finely chopped fresh basil.

YIELD: 7.3 oz zucchini noodles, 34 meatballs (1.13 oz each),
53 oz tomato ragout

| 1,200-CALORIE PLAN | 1,500-CALORIE PLAN | 1,800-CALORIE PLAN |
|---|---|---|
| ▶ 4 oz zucchini noodles + 6 meatballs + ¼ cup ragout | ▶ 8 oz zucchini noodles + 8 meatballs + ⅓ cup ragout | ▶ 8 oz zucchini noodles + 8 meatballs + ½ cup ragout |

# MEAL 6: SNACK P.M. 2:
### Hot Cocoa with Almond Milk

**INGREDIENTS**

- 1 cup sugar-free almond milk
- 1 tbsp unsweetened cocoa powder
- 2 stevia packets

**INSTRUCTIONS**

**1.** Heat the almond milk, cocoa, and stevia in a small pot over medium heat and bring to a boil. Remove from heat.

**2.** Blend, serve, and enjoy.

YIELD: 8 oz

| 1,200-CALORIE PLAN | 1,500-CALORIE PLAN | 1,800-CALORIE PLAN |
|---|---|---|
| ▶ 8 oz | ▶ Up to 16 oz | ▶ Up to 24 oz |

**DAY 10**

## Day 11

Visualize yourself, imagine yourself, see yourself as fabulous as you want to be. Cut the picture of a body you like from a magazine and stick your face on it. Put that image on your refrigerator, in your bathroom, or in any other place where you can always see it, especially when you feel like giving up.

## MEAL 1: PRE-WORKOUT SNACK:
### Egg Whites + Apple Green Tea Infusion

See Egg Whites recipe on page 91 and Apple Green Tea Infusion recipe on page 132.

## MEAL 2: BREAKFAST:
### Sweet Potato Tuna Croquettes

**INGREDIENTS**

1 egg white
½ red pepper
2 garlic cloves, crushed
cilantro to taste
1 cup tuna, well drained
1 cup sweet potatoes, mashed
½ cup almond flour
pink Himalayan sea salt to taste
pepper to taste
olive oil spray

**INSTRUCTIONS**

**1.** Mix egg white, red pepper, crushed garlic cloves, cilantro, tuna, sweet potato mash, and almond flour in a processor until you reach a smooth consistency. Add pink Himalayan sea salt and pepper to taste.

**2.** Transfer to an airtight container and refrigerate for 4 hours.

**3.** Wet your hands, shape the croquettes, and once they're ready, cook them in a nonstick skillet sprayed with olive oil, until they're brown. Then bake them in the oven at 325°F for 20 minutes. You can also use an air fryer to complete this step.

**4.** Serve and enjoy.

YIELD: 20 croquettes (1 oz each)

| 1,200-CALORIE PLAN | 1,500-CALORIE PLAN | 1,800-CALORIE PLAN |
|---|---|---|
| ▶ Up to 6 croquettes | ▶ Up to 9 croquettes | ▶ Up to 12 croquettes |

## MEAL 3: LUNCH:
**Chicken Curry + Brown Rice + Mixed Salad**

# chicken curry

**INGREDIENTS**

2 chicken breasts cut into ¾-inch cubes (16 oz)

½ cup nonfat Greek yogurt

2 garlic cloves, minced

1 tbsp garam masala or curry powder

2 tsps ginger, grated

½ tsp pepper flakes

olive oil spray

½ cup white onion, finely chopped

½ cup sweet peppers, finely chopped

1 hot pepper, finely chopped

¼ cup chives, finely chopped

½ cup celery, finely chopped

2 cups chicken broth or water

pink Himalayan sea salt to taste

pepper to taste

1 zucchini, finely chopped

1 cup cauliflower, chopped

¼ cup pickles, finely chopped

cilantro, chopped, to taste

**INSTRUCTIONS**

**1.** In a sealable container or bag mix the chicken with half the yogurt, the minced garlic, the garam masala or curry powder, the ginger, and the pepper flakes. Refrigerate for 12 hours.

**2.** Spray olive oil on a thick-bottomed pan and sauté the chicken until golden. Remove and set aside.

*(Recipe continues)*

DAY 11

**3.** To the same pot add a little more olive oil spray, and then add and sauté the chopped onions, peppers, chives, and celery.

**4.** Add the chicken and the chicken broth or water, and lower the heat to medium. When the broth is reduced by half and the consistency has become creamier, adjust the seasoning and add salt and pepper, and then add the remaining yogurt and the zucchini, cauliflower, and pickles.

**5.** Add chopped fresh cilantro and serve over a bed of Brown Rice.

YIELD: 21 oz

# brown rice

See recipe on page 140.

# mixed salad

See recipe on page 130.

| 1,200-CALORIE PLAN | 1,500-CALORIE PLAN | 1,800-CALORIE PLAN |
|---|---|---|
| ▶5 oz chicken curry + 2.1 oz brown rice + 1 bowl mixed salad | ▶6 oz chicken curry + 4.3 oz brown rice + 1 bowl mixed salad | ▶8.6 oz chicken curry + 6½ oz brown rice + 1 bowl mixed salad |

## MEAL 4: SNACK P.M. 1:
### Turkey, Tomato, and Lettuce Sandwich

**INGREDIENTS**

4 cabbage leaves
3 slices of turkey breast ham, low-fat
4 tomato slices, large
1 cup alfalfa sprouts
mustard to taste

**INSTRUCTIONS**

**1.** Take 2 cabbage leaves and, on top of them, place the turkey breast ham, the tomato slices, the alfalfa sprouts, and the mustard to taste.

**2.** Top with 2 more cabbage leaves and serve as a sandwich.

YIELD: 1 sandwich (4½ oz)

| 1,200-CALORIE PLAN | 1,500-CALORIE PLAN | 1,800-CALORIE PLAN |
|---|---|---|
| ▶½ sandwich | ▶1 sandwich | ▶1½ sandwiches |

DAY 11

# stuffed squid

**INGREDIENTS**

16 oz squid, washed and whole
olive oil spray
1 tbsp paprika
1 tbsp chili powder
16 oz shrimp, washed and deveined
½ cup onion, diced
½ cup leeks, chopped
½ cup celery, diced
½ red pepper, diced
1 tbsp garlic, crushed
pink Himalayan sea salt to taste
zest and juice of 1 lemon
1 tbsp fresh parsley, finely chopped

**INSTRUCTIONS**

**FOR THE FILLING**

**1.** Take the squid and remove the tentacles and lateral fins from the body and leave aside. Chop the tentacles and fins.

**2.** Heat a frying pan over high heat, spray it with olive oil, and add the paprika and chili powder. Then stir in the shrimp and the chopped pieces of squid. Remove from heat and reserve.

**3.** In the same skillet, sauté the onion, leeks, celery, peppers, and garlic. Cook for 5 minutes; season with salt, half of the lemon zest, and lemon juice; and add the chopped shrimp, squid, and parsley to the skillet.

**4.** Remove from heat and allow the filling to cool.

**STUFFING THE SQUID:**

**1.** Season the squid bodies with salt and the rest of the lemon zest.

**2.** Stuff each squid with the help of a teaspoon, without overstuffing. Close the squid's mouth with a toothpick.

**3.** Preheat the oven to 350° F.

*(Recipe continues)*

DAY 11

**4.** Spray a baking dish with olive oil and place the squid on it. Cook in the oven for approximately 10 minutes.

**5.** Take the squid out of the oven and remove the toothpicks very carefully. Serve with the Grilled Asparagus.

YIELD: 16 squids, each with 2½ oz filling

## grilled asparagus

See recipe on page 117.

| 1,200-CALORIE PLAN | 1,500-CALORIE PLAN | 1,800-CALORIE PLAN |
|---|---|---|
| ▶ 4 stuffed squid + 3.3–10 oz grilled asparagus | ▶ 5 stuffed squid + 3.3–10 oz grilled asparagus | ▶ 7 stuffed squid + 3.3–10 oz grilled asparagus |

## MEAL 6: SNACK P.M. 2:
**Vanilla Protein Pancakes**

### INGREDIENTS

2 egg whites
2 stevia packets
1 scoop of vanilla whey protein
½ tsp ground cinnamon
olive oil spray

### INSTRUCTIONS

**1.** With the help of an electric mixer at high speed, beat the egg whites until they form soft peaks.

**2.** Decrease the speed and slowly add the stevia, the whey protein, and the cinnamon.

**3.** Heat a nonstick pan, spray it with olive oil, and add half the mixture. Cover, and when the pancake starts to brown a little, flip it to cook on the other side.

**4.** Serve and enjoy.

YIELD: 2 pancakes (1½ oz each)

| 1,200-CALORIE PLAN | 1,500-CALORIE PLAN | 1,800-CALORIE PLAN |
|---|---|---|
| ▶ 1 pancake | ▶ 1 pancake | ▶ 2 pancakes |

DAY 11

# Day 12

When you feel like you are going to give up, remember those who made fun of you, criticized you, or didn't believe in you. Relive that emotion in detail and turn it into anger and strength to take on a heavier load, do another set, or increase your cardio.

Get your revenge!

## MEAL 1: PRE-WORKOUT SNACK:
### Egg Whites + Apple Green Tea Infusion

See Egg Whites recipe on page 91 and Apple Green Tea Infusion recipe on page 132.

## MEAL 2: BREAKFAST:
### Spanish Tortilla + *Criollo* Potatoes

**INGREDIENTS**

olive oil spray
2 medium-sized *criollo* potatoes, diced (2.65 oz)
2 tbsps purple onion, finely chopped
3 egg whites plus 1 egg yolk
pink Himalayan sea salt to taste
pepper to taste

**INSTRUCTIONS**

**1.** Heat a nonstick skillet over medium heat. Spray it with olive oil and sauté the diced potatoes until they are brown. Remove.

**2.** Add the purple onion and sauté for 2 minutes.

**3.** Add the eggs and salt and pepper to taste, and mix until the egg is fully cooked.

**4.** Serve and enjoy.

YIELD: 1 tortilla (5.6 oz)

| 1,200-CALORIE PLAN | 1,500-CALORIE PLAN | 1,800-CALORIE PLAN |
|---|---|---|
| ►1 tortilla (5.6 oz) | ►1½ tortillas (8.4 oz) | ►2 tortillas (11 oz) |

DAY 12

# grilled pork loin

### INGREDIENTS

½ pork loin (8 oz)
½ tsp paprika powder
½ tsp BBQ seasoning
1 tsp sriracha sauce
¼ cup red wine
olive oil spray
pink Himalayan sea salt to taste
pepper to taste

### INSTRUCTIONS

**1.** In a sealed plastic bag, marinate the pork loin along with the paprika, BBQ seasoning, sriracha sauce, and wine. Refrigerate for at least 4 hours.

**2.** Heat a frying pan or griddle over high heat and spray with the olive oil.

**3.** Add the pork loin to the skillet and sear it by carefully browning all sides.

**4.** Season to taste with salt and pepper.

**5.** Put the pan with the pork loin in the oven at 350°F and cook for 15 to 20 minutes. Take it out of the oven and let the pork loin sit for a little while before serving.

**6.** Enjoy.

YIELD: 14 oz

# brown rice

See recipe on page 140.

# steamed broccoli

See recipe on page 140.

| 1,200-CALORIE PLAN | 1,500-CALORIE PLAN | 1,800-CALORIE PLAN |
|---|---|---|
| ▶ 4 oz grilled pork loin + 2.1 oz brown rice + steamed broccoli | ▶ 5 oz grilled pork loin + 4.3 oz brown rice + steamed broccoli | ▶ 7 oz grilled pork loin + 6½ oz brown rice + steamed broccoli |

DAY 12

## MEAL 4: SNACK P.M. 1:
### Oatmeal Protein Cookies

**INGREDIENTS**

3 egg whites
1 cup rolled oats, uncooked
1 tbsp chia seeds
1 tbsp flaxseeds
¼ cup dates, diced
¼ cup blueberries, dehydrated and chopped
1 tsp cinnamon
1 tbsp coconut oil
2 tbsps coconut, grated, unsweetened
½ tbsp vanilla
1 scoop of vanilla whey protein
1 tsp baking soda
vegetable oil spray

**INSTRUCTIONS**

**1.** With the help of an electric mixer, beat 3 egg whites to form soft peaks.

**2.** Stop the mixer and manually add the rolled oats, chia seeds, flaxseeds, diced dates, blueberries, cinnamon, coconut oil, coconut, vanilla, vanilla whey protein, and baking soda.

**3.** Mix well with a spatula until you obtain a smooth dough.

**4.** Spray a little vegetable oil on a baking sheet and place a tablespoon of the dough on it, flattening it with the spatula to form a cookie.

**5.** Bake at 325°F for 20 minutes or until golden. Remove and allow to cool.

YIELD: 12 cookies (1 oz each)

| 1,200-CALORIE PLAN | 1,500-CALORIE PLAN | 1,800-CALORIE PLAN |
|---|---|---|
| ▶ 1 cookie | ▶ Up to 2 cookies | ▶ Up to 2½ cookies |

DAY 12

# MEAL 5: DINNER:

**Whitefish Ceviche**

**INGREDIENTS**

16 oz fresh whitefish fillets (corvina, dorado, or robalo)
1 purple onion, julienned
10 sweet cherry peppers, julienned
1 hot chili pepper, seeded and deveined, cut brunoise style
½ cup lemon juice
cilantro, finely chopped to taste
zest of 1 lemon
pink Himalayan sea salt to taste
pepper to taste

**INSTRUCTIONS**

**1.** Cut the whitefish fillets into ¾-inch cubes.

**2.** In a glass bowl, mix the fish with the vegetables and add the lemon juice, cilantro, lemon zest, and salt and pepper to taste.

**3.** Adjust the seasoning and refrigerate, covered with plastic film, for 5 minutes or until the fish turns white. Serve in a chilled glass bowl and enjoy.

**YIELD: 20 oz**

| 1,200-CALORIE PLAN | 1,500-CALORIE PLAN | 1,800-CALORIE PLAN |
|---|---|---|
| ►8½ oz | ►9.7 oz | ►12.6 oz |

# MEAL 6: SNACK P.M. 2:

**Turkey Stew with Spinach and Carrots**

**INGREDIENTS**

3.7 oz Turkey Stew (see recipe on page 131)
1 cup squash
½ cup carrots, grated
juice of 1 lemon
olive oil to taste
pink Himalayan sea salt to taste
pepper to taste

**DAY 12**

## INSTRUCTIONS

Mix the Turkey Stew, squash, and carrots and season with lemon, olive oil, and salt and pepper to taste.

YIELD: 1 cup

**1,200-CALORIE PLAN**
▶ 1 cup

**1,500-CALORIE PLAN**
▶ 1½ cups

**1,800-CALORIE PLAN**
▶ Up to 2 cups

## Day 13

*Why am I doing this?* Make your answer cheerful, fun, exciting ... If you feel excited about your destination, the journey will be so much easier. Always remember the list of reasons that led you to want to change some aspect of your body or your life.

## MEAL 1: PRE-WORKOUT SNACK:
**Egg Whites + Apple Green Tea Infusion**

See Egg Whites recipe on page 91 and Apple Green Tea Infusion recipe on page 132.

## MEAL 2: BREAKFAST:
**Chicken-and-Avocado-Filled Yucca Arepas**

## yucca arepas

### INGREDIENTS

1 cup cassava (7.05 oz), cooked and mashed
1 egg white
½ cup oat bran (2.55 oz)
1 tbsp chia seeds, flaxseeds, and hemp seeds
pink Himalayan sea salt to taste
pepper to taste
2–3 tbsps water
olive oil spray

### INSTRUCTIONS

**1.** In a bowl or in a food processor, mix the mashed yucca with the egg white, oat bran, chia seeds, flaxseeds, hemp seeds, salt, pepper, and water. If the dough becomes too tough, add more water.

**2.** Knead well until the dough feels smooth like clay yet firm enough to shape into arepas.

**3.** With wet hands, take portions of the dough and make balls. Flatten them slightly to make arepas.

**4.** Heat a frying pan or griddle and spray it with olive oil. Cook the arepas until they are brown on both sides, and then put them in the oven at 350°F for 25 minutes to finish cooking them. If you have an air fryer, you can use that instead of the oven.

**THE HOT BODY DIET**

DAY 13

**5.** Serve and enjoy.

YIELD: 6 arepas (4.58 oz each)

# chicken and avocado filling

### INGREDIENTS

    1 cup chicken, cooked and shredded
    1 Hass avocado (4.55 oz)
    1 tbsp onion, finely chopped
    1 bunch of cilantro
    pink Himalayan sea salt to taste
    pepper to taste

### INSTRUCTIONS

With the help of a fork, mix all the ingredients until you have a uniform paste that you can use to fill the arepa.

YIELD: 10½ oz

| 1,200-CALORIE PLAN | 1,500-CALORIE PLAN | 1,800-CALORIE PLAN |
|---|---|---|
| ▶1 arepa + 3½ oz chicken and avocado filling | ▶1½ arepas + 5 oz chicken and avocado filling | ▶2 arepas + 7 oz chicken and avocado filling |

## MEAL 3: LUNCH:
**Chicken Breast + Baked Sweet Potato Fries + Grilled Vegetable Kebabs**

# chicken breast

### INGREDIENTS

    1 tbsp BBQ seasoning
    1 tsp paprika
    1 tsp chili powder
    pink Himalayan sea salt to taste
    2 whole chicken breast fillets, with skin and bone (16 oz)
    1 garlic clove, crushed
    juice and zest of 1 lemon

*(Recipe continues)*

**DAY 13**

## INSTRUCTIONS

**1.** In a small cup, combine the BBQ seasoning, paprika, chili powder, and salt.

**2.** In a sealed plastic bag, marinate the chicken with the spices, garlic, lemon juice, lemon zest, and salt. Refrigerate for 3 hours.

**3.** Heat the griddle or grill to high heat to roast the chicken, making sure it browns on all sides. When you have reached the desired degree of doneness, remove from the heat and let stand before serving accompanied by Baked Sweet Potato Fries and a Grilled Vegetable Kebab.

YIELD: 14 oz cooked breast

# baked sweet potato fries

## INGREDIENTS

2 sweet potatoes, washed and scrubbed
1 bunch fresh parsley, chopped
pink Himalayan sea salt to taste
pepper to taste
olive oil spray

## INSTRUCTIONS

**1.** Cut the raw sweet potatoes into sticks and place them on a nonstick baking sheet or perforated tray.

**2.** Season with parsley, salt, and pepper and spray with the olive oil.

**3.** Put them in a preheated oven at 350°F for 30 minutes, ensuring that they do not burn.

**4.** When they start to brown on one side, flip them over. Remove from the oven and serve. You can also make them in an air fryer if you have one.

YIELD: 24 oz baked sweet potato

# grilled vegetable kebabs

## INGREDIENTS

wooden skewers
1 white onion, quartered
1 red pepper, diced
1 green pepper, diced
1 yellow pepper, diced
1 cup mushrooms, whole
1 cup zucchini, diced

1 cup cherry tomatoes
½ tbsp paprika
pink Himalayan sea salt to taste
freshly ground black pepper to taste
olive oil spray

## INSTRUCTIONS

**1.** Moisten the skewers to prevent them from burning.

**2.** Assemble the kebabs by mixing the vegetables to taste on the skewers, and season with paprika, salt, and pepper.

**3.** Fire up a grill or heat a griddle and spray the skewers with olive oil. Turn them from time to time as you cook them, making sure they cook on all sides.

YIELD: 8 skewers (3 oz each)

| 1,200-CALORIE PLAN | 1,500-CALORIE PLAN | 1,800-CALORIE PLAN |
|---|---|---|
| ▶ 4 oz chicken breast + 2.1 oz baked sweet potato fries + 1 grilled vegetable kebab | ▶ 5 oz chicken breast + 4.3 oz baked sweet potato fries + up to 2 grilled vegetable kebabs | ▶ 7 oz chicken breast + 6½ oz baked sweet potato fries + up to 3 grilled vegetable kebabs |

# MEAL 4: SNACK P.M. 1:
### Strawberry Protein Shake

## INGREDIENTS

1 cup almond milk
½ cup frozen strawberries
1 tsp chia seeds
1 tsp ground flaxseeds
2 stevia packets
zest of ½ lemon
1 spearmint leaf, for garnish

## INSTRUCTIONS

**1.** Mix all ingredients except the spearment leaf in a blender for 1 minute. Garnish with the spearmint leaf.

**2.** Serve and enjoy.

YIELD: 1 cup (16 oz)

| 1,200-CALORIE PLAN | 1,500-CALORIE PLAN | 1,800-CALORIE PLAN |
|---|---|---|
| ▶ 12 oz | ▶ Up to 16 oz | ▶ Up to 20 oz |

DAY 13

# tuna, avocado, cucumber, and wakame roll

**INGREDIENTS**

1 large Japanese cucumber
2 sheets of nori
4 oz red tuna cut into strips 1 cm thick
¼ cup wakame
1 Hass avocado, thinly sliced

**INSTRUCTIONS**

**1.** Use a sharp knife to slice the cucumber lengthwise (not in rounds) into thin slices. Reserve.

**2.** Take a sushi mat and wrap it in baking paper. Place the cucumber slices on the mat, forming a first layer, and on top of it place a sheet of nori to make the roll sturdy.

**3.** Fill the roll with the red tuna, wakame, and avocado slices, all well placed on the top third of the roll.

**4.** Use the bamboo mat to shape the roll, and once you are done, make sure it is properly sealed. Close the roll and press firmly until it becomes compact. Remove the bamboo mat and cut the roll into pieces using a sharp knife, moistening the blade after every cut in order to prevent the roll from sticking or breaking apart.

**YIELD: 2 rolls**

# ponzu sauce

**INGREDIENTS**

½ cup lemon juice
¼ cup orange juice
¾ cup light soy sauce
1 tbsp rice vinegar
1 tbsp rice wine (mirin)

**INSTRUCTIONS**

In a large bowl, whisk together all the ingredients until they are fully mixed.

DAY 13

## MEAL 3: LUNCH:

**Beef Tenderloin Kebabs + Baked *Criollo* Potatoes + Pineapple Coleslaw Salad**

### INGREDIENTS

rosemary branches or wooden skewers
16 oz beef tenderloin, cleaned and cut in cubes
1 onion, quartered
1 red pepper, cut in cubes
1 green pepper, cut in cubes
1 yellow pepper, cut in cubes
10 mushrooms, whole
10 cherry tomatoes
1 tbsp BBQ seasoning
1 tbsp paprika powder
1 tbsp garlic, crushed
pink Himalayan sea salt to taste
freshly ground pepper to taste
olive oil spray

### INSTRUCTIONS

**1.** If you are using rosemary sticks, remove the leaves, leaving only the tops. With the help of a sharp knife, clean the stems and cut the tips to be able to prick. If you do not have rosemary sticks, moisten the wooden skewers.

**2.** Assemble the kebabs as follows: beef, onion, red pepper, beef, green pepper, onion, yellow pepper, onion, beef, and so on until you complete the desired pattern, finishing off with a cherry tomato to close the skewer.

**3.** Season the kebabs with the BBQ seasoning, paprika powder, crushed garlic, salt, pepper, and olive oil spray.

**4.** Fire up a grill, or heat a griddle to high and spray it with olive oil. Place the kebabs on the grill or griddle and cook them for 5 minutes on each side or until the desired degree of doneness is achieved. Remove them from the grill or griddle and and serve with Baked *Criollo* Potatoes.

**YIELD: 6 kebabs**

DAY 14

# baked *criollo* potatoes

**INGREDIENTS**

3½ oz *criollo* potatoes
olive oil spray
1 tbsp garlic, crushed
fresh parsley, chopped
pink Himalayan sea salt to taste
pepper to taste

**INSTRUCTIONS**

**1.** Wash, scrub, and dry the potatoes; you can leave the skin on. Quarter each potato lengthwise, and spray with olive oil.

**2.** Season with the crushed garlic, parsley, and salt and pepper to taste. Transfer to a baking dish and bake at 350°F for 25 to 30 minutes, until golden brown.

**YIELD: 3½ baked potatoes**

# pineapple coleslaw salad

**INGREDIENTS**

½ pineapple, peeled
1 tbsp paprika
½ tbsp five-spices seasoning
½ cup fat-free Greek yogurt
1 tbsp apple cider vinegar
1 tbsp lemon juice
½ tsp mustard
2 stevia packets
pink Himalayan sea salt to taste
freshly ground fresh pepper to taste
zest of 1 lemon
2 cups white cabbage, finely chopped
1 cup purple cabbage, finely chopped
½ cup carrot, thinly grated
chives, finely cut

**INSTRUCTIONS**

**1.** Season the pineapple with paprika and five-spices seasoning. It can be cut into disks for easy grilling and seasoning.

**2.** Grill the pineapple on a grill or griddle, being careful not to burn it. Once it's fully grilled, remove it, cut it into small cubes, and set it aside.

**3.** In a large stainless steel bowl, whisk together the yogurt, vinegar, lemon juice, mustard, and stevia to make the dressing.

**4.** Pour the dressing over the grilled pineapple and season with salt and pepper to taste. Add lemon zest and set aside.

**5.** In a large salad bowl, mix the cabbages, carrots, and dressing. Sprinkle with fresh chives before serving.

YIELD: 4 cups of salad

| 1,200-CALORIE PLAN | 1,500-CALORIE PLAN | 1,800-CALORIE PLAN |
|---|---|---|
| ▶ 1½ beef tenderloin kebabs + 2.6 oz *criollo* potatoes + 1 cup pineapple coleslaw salad | ▶ 2 beef tenderloin kebabs + 5.3 oz *criollo* potatoes + 1 cup pineapple coleslaw salad | ▶ Up to 3 beef tenderloin kebabs + 8 oz *criollo* potatoes + 1 cup pineapple coleslaw salad |

## MEAL 4: SNACK P.M. 1:
### Protein Greek Yogurt with Berries

**INGREDIENTS**

1 cup Greek yogurt
½ scoop of vanilla whey protein
½ tsp vanilla extract
juice of ½ lemon
1 stevia packet
zest of 1 lemon
½ cup chopped berries (strawberries, blackberries, blueberries, and raspberries)

**INSTRUCTIONS**

**1.** Whisk all ingredients together.

**2.** Serve and enjoy.

YIELD: 9 oz yogurt + 3 oz berries

| 1,200-CALORIE PLAN | 1,500-CALORIE PLAN | 1,800-CALORIE PLAN |
|---|---|---|
| ▶ ½ cup Greek yogurt + 1½ oz berries | ▶ ½ cup Greek yogurt + 1½ oz berries | ▶ ¾ cup Greek yogurt + 2 oz berries |

DAY 14

# turkey ragout

**INGREDIENTS**

- 1 cup white onion, diced
- ¼ cup chives
- ¼ cup celery, chopped
- ¼ cup garlic, chopped
- ½ cup sweet peppers, chopped
- 1 tbsp water
- olive oil spray
- Italian spices (oregano, sage, thyme, and rosemary) to taste
- 16 oz ground turkey
- pink Himalayan sea salt to taste
- pepper to taste
- ½ cup red pepper, chopped
- 4 garlic cloves, roasted
- 4 cups tomatoes, peeled and seeded
- 8 fresh basil leaves
- 1 tbsp balsamic vinegar
- 2 tbsps tomato paste
- 1 stevia packet
- 1 bay leaf
- 1 tsp Dijon mustard

**INSTRUCTIONS**

**1.** In a blender, process the onion, chives, celery, garlic, sweet peppers, and water until you obtain a smooth paste.

**2.** Spray a frying pan with olive oil and add the Italian spices (oregano, sage, thyme, and rosemary) and ground turkey.

**3.** Break apart and cook the ground turkey until it is brown and fully cooked. Season with salt and pepper.

**4.** Add the blended vegetable mix to the turkey and sauté over medium heat.

**5.** In the blender, process the red pepper, garlic, tomatoes, and basil for one minute until you obtain a homogenous liquid. Add it to the ground turkey in the pan, lower the heat to a simmer, and cook uncovered for about 40 minutes.

DAY 14

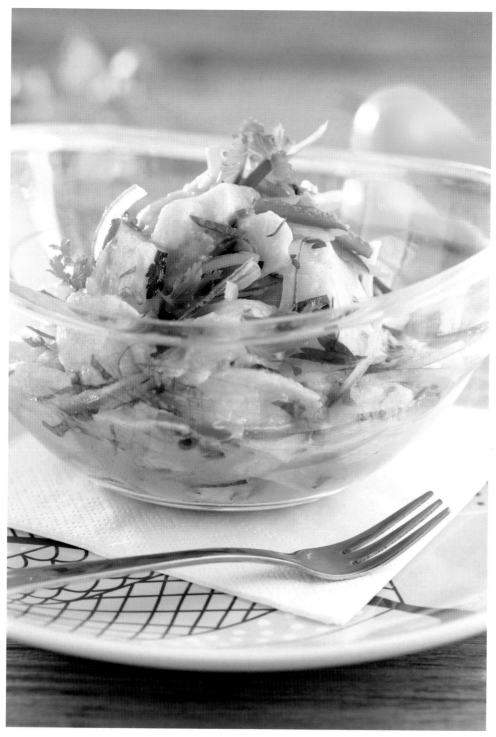

*Whitefish Ceviche*

All photographs are courtesy of Angel Rodriguez, unless otherwise noted.

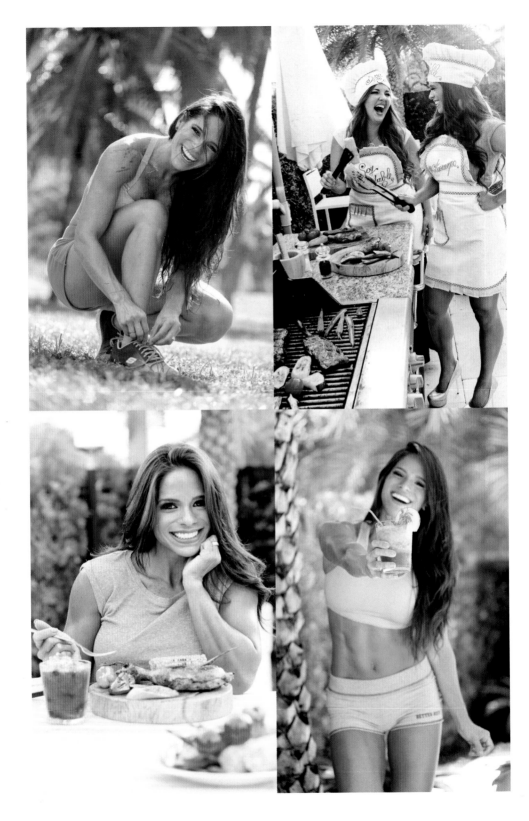

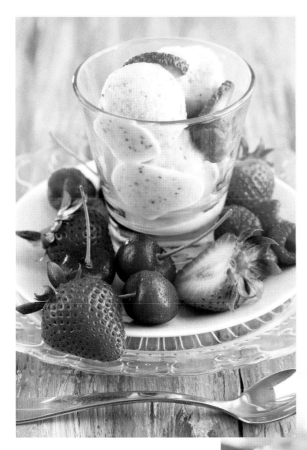
*Berry Protein Ice Cream*

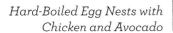
*Hard-Boiled Egg Nests with
Chicken and Avocado*

*Grilled Sirloin Steak*

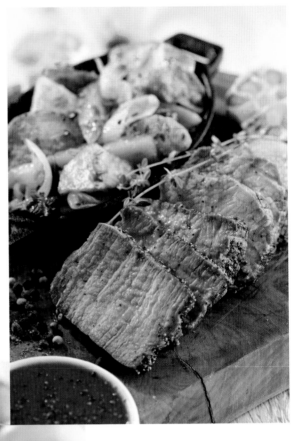

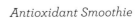
*Antioxidant Smoothie*

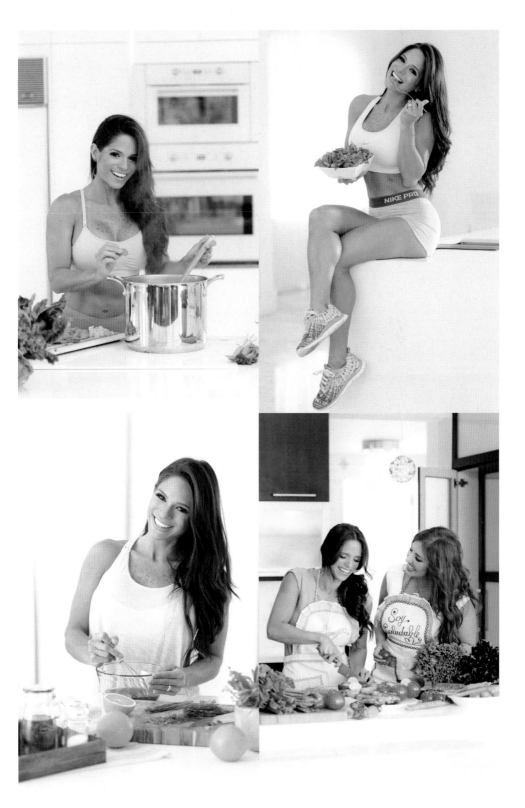

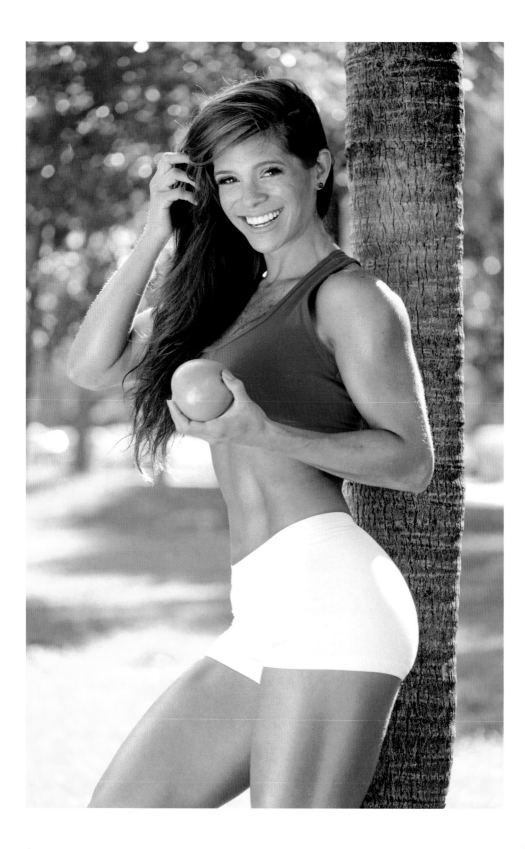

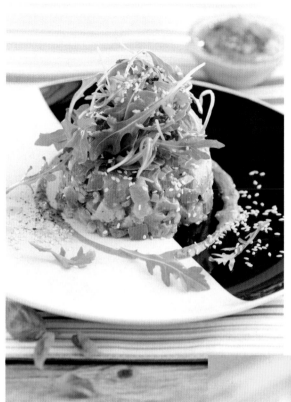

*Tuna Avocado Tartar*

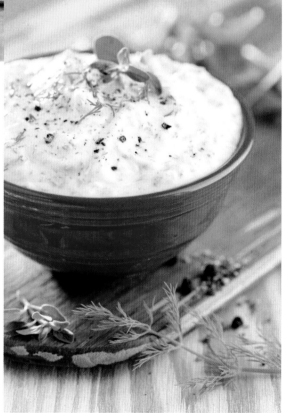

*Tzatziki*

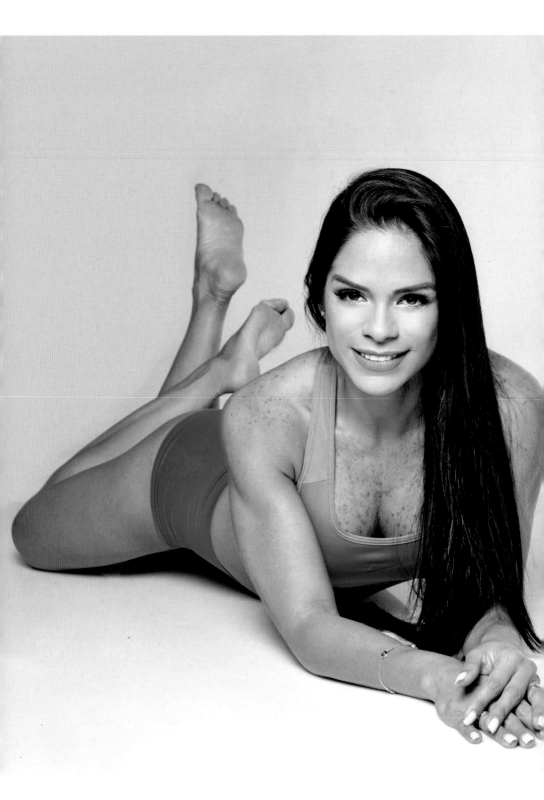

Photograph courtesy of Ruben Dario.

**6.** Add the balsamic vinegar, tomato paste, stevia, bay leaf, and mustard to the sauce. Allow almost all the liquid to reduce until you obtain the desired consistency.

**7.** Adjust the seasoning with salt and pepper and remove from the heat. Set aside.

# zucchini cannelloni

### INGREDIENTS

4 large zucchini
olive oil spray
1 cup vegetarian cheese (almond cheese), shredded
6 large basil leaves for garnish

### INSTRUCTIONS

**1.** Using a mandoline or a sharp knife, cut the zucchini lengthwise into slices.

**2.** Fire up a grill or griddle over high heat, spray it with olive oil, and quickly sear the zucchini slices on all sides.

**3.** In a baking dish sprayed with olive oil, assemble the cannelloni by wrapping each zucchini slice around 1 tablespoon of Turkey Ragout (it should be cold to facilitate assembly). Place the cannelloni in rows on a tray until it is completely full. Sprinkle the grated almond cheese over the cannelloni.

**4.** Heat the oven to 350°F and bake the tray of cannelloni for 8 to 10 minutes. Remove the tray from the oven when the cannelloni look golden and garnish with basil leaves.

YIELD: 30 cannelloni (1.6 oz each)

| 1,200-CALORIE PLAN | 1,500-CALORIE PLAN | 1,800-CALORIE PLAN |
|---|---|---|
| ▶ 4 cannelloni | ▶ 5 cannelloni | ▶ Up to 7 cannelloni |

DAY 14

## MEAL 6: SNACK P.M. 2:
### Kiwi or Berries with Fat-Free Whipped Cream

**INGREDIENTS**

1 cup berries (raspberries, blackberries, or blueberries) or kiwi

4 tbsps whipped cream, sugar-free

**INSTRUCTIONS**

Serve the berries or kiwi in a bowl and top with sugar-free whipped cream.

| 1,200-CALORIE PLAN | 1,500-CALORIE PLAN | 1,800-CALORIE PLAN |
|---|---|---|
| ►1 cup berries or kiwi + 4 tbsps whipped cream | ►Up to 1½ cups berries or kiwi + 4 tbsps whipped cream | ►Up to 2 cups berries or kiwi + 4 tbsps whipped cream |

DAY 14

## greek yogurt with vanilla protein

**INGREDIENTS**

1 cup Greek yogurt
½ scoop of vanilla whey protein
1 stevia packet
½ tsp vanilla
zest of 1 lemon (optional)

**INSTRUCTIONS**

**1.** In a medium bowl, whisk together the Greek yogurt, whey protein, stevia, and vanilla.

**2.** If desired, add lemon zest before serving.

YIELD: 1 cup (8½ oz)

### Prepare It in 10 Different Flavors

Add ingredients to each yogurt cup:

1. **Chocolate:** Replace the vanilla whey protein with chocolate whey protein and add 1 teaspoon of sugar-free cocoa powder.
2. **Lemon:** Add the zest of ½ lemon and the juice of 1 lemon.
3. **Cinnamon:** Add 1 teaspoon of cinnamon and 1 teaspoon of sliced almonds.
4. **Marbled:** Divide the mixture into two equal parts. Add cocoa powder and unsweetened chocolate chips to one of the halves to decorate.
5. **Walnut Raisin:** Add 1 tablespoon of raisins, a fistful of chopped walnuts, and a pinch of cinnamon.
6. **Berries:** Add ½ cup of several different berries (strawberries, blueberries, raspberries, or blackberries).
7. **Granola:** Add ⅓ cup of granola containing less than 5 grams of sugar.

8. **Acai Berry**: Add 1 tablespoon of acai berry powder.
9. **Piña Colada**: Add pieces of fresh pineapple, 1 tablespoon of grated sugar-free coconut, and a few drops of coconut essence.
10. **Mango**: Add half a ripe mango, diced.

## Day 15

Don't let anything or anyone sabotage your effort. Think about how good you're going to feel when you get rid of the fat and the extra inches. Don't fool yourself. Don't waste your time, your effort, or your money. Keep going—if I was able to do it, why can't you?

## MEAL 1: PRE-WORKOUT SNACK:
**Egg Whites + Antioxidant Smoothie**

See Egg Whites recipe on page 91.

# antioxidant smoothie

**INGREDIENTS**

1 cup water or sugar-free almond milk
1 scoop of vanilla or chocolate whey protein
½ cup berries (strawberries, blackberries, raspberries, or blueberries)
1 tbsp acai berry powder (optional)
2 stevia packets

**INSTRUCTIONS**

1. Mix all ingredients in a blender and process for 1 minute.
2. Serve and enjoy.

YIELD: 1 cup (16 oz)

| 1,200-CALORIE PLAN | 1,500-CALORIE PLAN | 1,800-CALORIE PLAN |
|---|---|---|
| ►8 oz | ►12 oz | ►16 oz |

## MEAL 2: BREAKFAST:
**Walnut Raisin Protein Waffles**

### INGREDIENTS

⅓ cup oats (1.2 oz)

2 egg whites

¼ cup walnuts

1 tbsp raisins

1 scoop of vanilla whey protein

⅓ cup almond milk

½ tsp cinnamon

1 packet of stevia

vegetable oil spray

maple syrup (sugar free)

### INSTRUCTIONS

**1.** In a blender, blend the oats, egg whites, walnuts, raisins, whey protein, almond milk, cinnamon, and stevia for 1 minute.

**2.** Heat a waffle pan and spray it with vegetable oil. Pour half the mixture into the waffle pan and close it. Once the waffle turns golden (or the light on the waffle pan changes from red to green), remove it.

**3.** Serve with sugar-free maple syrup and enjoy!

YIELD: 2 waffles (2.1 oz each)

| 1,200-CALORIE PLAN | 1,500-CALORIE PLAN | 1,800-CALORIE PLAN |
|---|---|---|
| ▶ 1 waffle | ▶ 1½ waffles | ▶ 2 waffles |

## MEAL 3: LUNCH:
**Baked Pork Loin + Waldorf Salad**

# baked pork loin

### INGREDIENTS

16 oz pork loin

zest of 1 orange

1 cup orange juice

2 tbsps mix of herbs and spices (rosemary, thyme, oregano, garlic, sage, curry, tarragon, pepper, cumin, ginger, basil, red pepper flakes, fennel seeds, sesame, coriander, or mustard), crushed in a mortar, to taste

¼ cup red wine
vegetable oil spray

## INSTRUCTIONS

**1.** In a sealed plastic bag, marinate the pork loin with the orange juice and orange zest and refrigerate for 8 hours.

**2.** Drain the pork well and place it on top of a board covered with the mix of ground spices. Turn it until all parts are covered.

**3.** Place a nonstick pan or iron skillet over high heat and spray it with vegetable oil. When it becomes very hot, add the pork loin and sear it on all sides.

**4.** Finish cooking in the oven, placing the pork loin and the red wine in a covered baking dish for 20 minutes at 350°F.

**5.** Uncover and cook for another 25 minutes or until golden.

**6.** Slice and serve immediately.

YIELD: 14 oz

# waldorf salad

## INGREDIENTS

FOR THE DRESSING
½ cup fat-free Greek yogurt
¼ cup apple cider vinegar
1 tbsp Dijon mustard
2 tbsps olive oil
2 stevia packets
pink Himalayan sea salt to taste
pepper to taste

FOR THE SALAD
2 cups lettuce, finely chopped
1 green apple, julienned
1 cup celery, julienned
½ cup walnuts, chopped
¼ cup raisins

## INSTRUCTIONS

**1.** In a bowl, prepare the dressing by whisking together the yogurt, vinegar, mustard, olive oil, and stevia. Season with salt and pepper to taste. Set aside in the refrigerator.

*(Recipe continues)*

DAY 15

**2.** Place all salad ingredients in a large salad bowl, add the dressing, and mix well.

**3.** Serve and enjoy.

YIELD: 3 cups salad

| 1,200-CALORIE PLAN | 1,500-CALORIE PLAN | 1,800-CALORIE PLAN |
|---|---|---|
| ▶ 4 oz baked pork loin + 1 cup Waldorf salad | ▶ 5 oz baked pork loin + 1 cup Waldorf salad | ▶ 7 oz baked pork loin + 1 cup Waldorf salad |

## MEAL 4: SNACK P.M. 1:
### Chocolate Fudge Fit Protein Cupcake

See recipe on page 89.

| 1,200-CALORIE PLAN | 1,500-CALORIE PLAN | 1,800-CALORIE PLAN |
|---|---|---|
| ▶ ½ cupcake | ▶ 1 cupcake | ▶ 1 cupcake* <br> *You can eat a maximum of 1½ cupcakes. |

## MEAL 5: DINNER:
### Chicken and Vegetable Noodle Ramen Soup

**INGREDIENTS**

1 chicken thigh fillet, diced (4 oz)
½ tsp ginger, grated
zest of 1 lemon
2 tbsps light soy sauce
coconut oil spray
¼ cup red pepper, finely chopped
¼ cup onion, thinly sliced
¼ cup sweet peppers, finely chopped
1 hot pepper (jalapeño, rocoto, or habanero), thinly sliced
¼ cup baby carrots, julienned
¼ cup baby zucchini, julienned
¼ cup mushrooms, quartered
1 asparagus spear, chopped
¼ cup broccoli, chopped
1½ cups chicken broth
pink Himalayan sea salt
pepper

DAY 15

1 tbsp sriracha sauce

1 egg

½ cup bean sprouts

2½ oz brown rice noodles

1 tsp fresh cilantro, chopped

1 tsp chives, finely chopped

**INSTRUCTIONS**

**1.** Place the chicken in a bowl and season it with ginger, lemon zest, and soy sauce.

**2.** In a wide nonstick skillet or wok over high heat and sprayed with coconut oil, place the chicken and toss it until golden. Set aside.

**3.** Lower the heat to medium, gradually add the vegetables to the same skillet and sauté for 1 minute, in order to keep them crunchy.

**4.** Turn up the heat and add the chicken. Immediately add the chicken broth and lower the heat to a simmer. Adjust the seasoning with salt, pepper, and the sriracha sauce.

**5.** Add the egg, bean sprouts, and rice noodles. Allow them to cook for a couple of minutes, and then turn off the heat. Serve in a bowl and add chopped cilantro and fresh chives.

**YIELD: 1 ramen bowl (13.3 oz)**

| 1,200-CALORIE PLAN | 1,500-CALORIE PLAN | 1,800-CALORIE PLAN |
|---|---|---|
| ▶ 10 oz | ▶ 13.3 oz | ▶ 16.6 oz |

## MEAL 6: SNACK P.M. 2:
### Baked Pork Loin

See recipe on page 176.

| 1,200-CALORIE PLAN | 1,500-CALORIE PLAN | 1,800-CALORIE PLAN |
|---|---|---|
| ▶ 2½ oz | ▶ 3½ oz | ▶ 4½ oz |

DAY 15

## Day 16

Stay away from pessimists and critics—they are vampires who steal your energy. Get them out of your life and don't listen to them, because they have nothing valuable to add. You are on a path to strength and beauty. This is your place.

### MEAL 1: PRE-WORKOUT SNACK:
**Egg Whites + Antioxidant Smoothie**

See Egg Whites recipe on page 91 and Antioxidant Smoothie recipe on page 175.

### MEAL 2: BREAKFAST:
**Smoked Salmon Muffins + Sweet Potato and Beet Chips**

## smoked salmon muffins

**INGREDIENTS**

1 egg plus 3 egg whites
2 slices of smoked salmon, chopped (40 g)
1 sprig of fresh dill
½ tsp garlic, crushed
1 tbsp vegetarian mozzarella cheese

**INSTRUCTIONS**

1. Mix the eggs, salmon, dill, garlic, and mozzarella cheese with a fork.
2. Pour the mixture into a silicone muffin tray.
3. Bake for 20 minutes or until golden brown.
4. Serve and enjoy.

**YIELD: 3 muffins (2.4 oz each)**

DAY 16

# sweet potato and beet chips

**INGREDIENTS**

1 large sweet potato
1 large beet
pink Himalayan sea salt to taste
pepper to taste
1 tsp ground oregano
olive oil spray

**INSTRUCTIONS**

**1.** Peel the sweet potato and the beet with a potato peeler or sharp knife.

**2.** With the help of a mandoline or a wide-bladed knife, cut the potatato and the beet into thin sheets.

**3.** Season with salt, pepper, and oregano.

**4.** Place the sweet potato and beet slices on a perforated nonstick pan and spray them with olive oil.

**5.** Bake them for 30 minutes at low temperature (about 280°F), keeping an eye on them so they don't burn. Once they're golden on one side, flip them to cook the other. Remove them from the oven, serve, and enjoy.

**YIELD: 1.6 oz sweet potato chips + 1.3 oz beet chips**

**1,200-CALORIE PLAN**
▶ 2 muffins + 0.8 oz sweet potato chips + 0.6 oz beet chips

**1,500-CALORIE PLAN**
▶ 2½ muffins + 1.6 oz sweet potato chips + 1.3 oz beet chips

**1,800-CALORIE PLAN**
▶ 3½ muffins + 2½ oz sweet potato chips + 2 oz beet chips

DAY 16

# pepper steak

**INGREDIENTS**

16 oz beef tenderloin
pink Himalayan sea salt to taste
olive oil spray
1 tbsp freshly ground black, pink, white, and green pepper
mix of spices and dried herbs (oregano, sage, thyme, rosemary, red
    pepper flakes, peppercorns, bay leaves, and *guayabita* or jamaica
    pepper), crushed in a mortar

**INSTRUCTIONS**

**1.** Season the meat with salt and spray it with olive oil for the crust to adhere. Roll the whole piece of meat in the mix of peppers and crushed spices and herbs, covering completely.

**2.** In a frying pan, grill, or griddle on high heat, place the tenderloin and make sure to sear it on all sides.

**3.** Transfer it to a baking dish and bake at 350°F to finish cooking. Once you have reached the desired degree of doneness, remove it from the oven and let it stand for 5 to 10 minutes before slicing to serve and enjoy.

**YIELD: 13.3 oz**

# baked yucca chips

**INGREDIENTS**

7 oz yucca
pink Himalayan sea salt to taste
pepper to taste
1 tsp oregano
olive oil spray

**INSTRUCTIONS**

**1.** With the help of a mandoline or a sharp knife, cut the raw yucca into thin slices.

**2.** Season with salt, pepper, and oregano.

**3.** In a perforated nonstick pan place the yucca slices and spray them with oil spray.

DAY 16

**4.** Bake for 30 minutes at low temperature (about 280°F), keeping an eye on them so they don't burn. Once they're golden on one side, flip them to cook on the other. Remove them from the oven and serve them as a side.

YIELD: 1.3 oz yucca chips

## mixed salad

See recipe on page 130.

| 1,200-CALORIE PLAN | 1,500-CALORIE PLAN | 1,800-CALORIE PLAN |
|---|---|---|
| ▶ 4 oz pepper steak + 1.3 oz baked yucca chips + 1 cup mixed salad | ▶ 5 oz pepper steak + 2.6 oz baked yucca chips + 1 cup mixed salad | ▶ 7 oz pepper steak + 3.9 oz baked yucca chips + 2 cups mixed salad |

## MEAL 4: SNACK P.M. 1:
### Chicken, Cucumber, and Tomato Salad with Lemon

**INGREDIENTS**

4 oz chicken breast
1 garlic clove, crushed
salt to taste
oregano to taste
pepper to taste
1 cup spinach or mixed greens
½ cucumber, diced
1 medium tomato, diced
1 tsp olive oil
juice of 2 lemons

**INSTRUCTIONS**

**1.** Season the chicken breast with garlic, salt, oregano, and pepper, and grill until golden. Cut into cubes.

**2.** Mix all the vegetables in a salad bowl. Top with the chicken.

**3.** Garnish with olive oil, lemon, salt, and pepper. Serve and enjoy.

YIELD: 11½ oz

| 1,200-CALORIE PLAN | 1,500-CALORIE PLAN | 1,800-CALORIE PLAN |
|---|---|---|
| ▶ 5.8 oz | ▶ 9½ oz | ▶ 11½ oz |

DAY 16

## MEAL 5: DINNER:
**Turkey Portobello Burger**

**INGREDIENTS**

4 large portobello mushrooms

olive oil spray

2 grilled Turkey Patties (see recipe below)

¼ cup romaine lettuce

1 tomato, sliced

1 pickle, sliced

¼ cup onions, thinly sliced

¼ alfalfa sprouts

1 tbsp Dijon mustard

**INSTRUCTIONS**

**1.** Wash and wipe the portobellos with a damp cloth. Remove the stems, and use a teaspoon to remove the brown gills from the insides of the mushrooms.

**2.** Fire up the grill, or heat a nonstick skillet over high heat and spray it with olive oil, and quickly sear the portobellos on both sides.

**3.** After grilling the portobellos, place them stem side up and add one Turkey Patty, lettuce, tomato, pickles, onions, alfalfa sprouts, and mustard. Top the burger with another grilled portobello.

**4.** Serve and enjoy.

# turkey patty

**INGREDIENTS**

¼ cup red pepper, washed and deveined

¼ cup onion, chopped

2 egg whites

7½ oz lean ground turkey

pink Himalayan sea salt to taste

pepper to taste

2 tbsps ground almonds

olive oil spray

1 cup spinach leaves

**INSTRUCTIONS**

**1.** In a food processor, blend the peppers, onion, and egg whites until you obtain a homogenous mix. Reserve in a container.

**2.** Use the same processor to process the ground turkey, seasoned with salt and pepper. Add the vegetable mix, and then incorporate the almonds. Mix well.

**3.** Add salt and pepper to taste, and make patties weighing 3½ oz per serving.

**4.** Shape into hamburger patties and cook them on a nonstick skillet sprayed with olive oil until they brown. Serve and enjoy.

YIELD: 2 portobello burgers (6 oz each)

| 1,200-CALORIE PLAN | 1,500-CALORIE PLAN | 1,800-CALORIE PLAN |
|---|---|---|
| ▶ 1 portobello burger | ▶ 1½ portobello burgers | ▶ 2 portobello burgers |

## MEAL 6: SNACK P.M. 2:
### Apple Cinnamon Protein Shake

**INGREDIENTS**

1 cup sugar-free almond milk
½ apple, red or green, peeled
1 tsp ground cinnamon
1 scoop of vanilla whey protein

**INSTRUCTIONS**

Mix all ingredients. Serve and enjoy.

YIELD: 1 glass (9 oz)

| 1,200-CALORIE PLAN | 1,500-CALORIE PLAN | 1,800-CALORIE PLAN |
|---|---|---|
| ▶ 5 oz | ▶ 7 oz | ▶ 9 oz |

DAY 16

# Day 17

What makes you different from everyone else is that you forge ahead even when you think you can't go another step. If it were so easy to change what we do not like about our bodies and our lives, everyone would do it. But you will succeed, because you have decided not to abandon this path, no matter what happens.

## MEAL 1: PRE-WORKOUT SNACK:
### Egg Whites + Antioxidant Smoothie

See Egg Whites recipe on page 91 and Antioxidant Smoothie recipe on page 175.

## MEAL 2: BREAKFAST:
### Carrot Protein Pancakes

**INGREDIENTS**

⅓ cup rolled oats
1 egg plus 2 egg whites
½ scoop vanilla whey protein
¼ cup carrot, grated
1 tsp cinnamon
¼ tsp cloves
¼ tsp nutmeg
1 tsp stevia
½ tsp baking powder
1 or 2 tbsps almond milk or water
olive oil spray

**INSTRUCTIONS**

**1.** Mix all ingredients except the olive oil spray in a blender.

**2.** Spray a nonstick skillet with olive oil, heat it over medium heat, and add a portion of the mixture.

**3.** Cover the skillet. When the pancake begins to brown, flip it to cook on the other side. Serve and enjoy.

**YIELD: 5 pancakes (1.3 oz each)**

DAY 17

## MEAL 3: LUNCH:
**Baked Chicken + Pumpkin Puree + Green Salad**

# baked chicken

### INGREDIENTS

1 whole chicken, bone-in, no skin
5 sprigs of fresh thyme, plus more for seasoning
1 tsp fresh oregano, plus more for seasoning
1 tbsp Dijon mustard
¼ cup red wine
juice of 1 orange
1 white onion, grated
½ garlic head, cut lengthwise
1 leek, chopped
1 red pepper, julienned
1 onion, julienned
1 celery stem, chopped
olive oil spray
zest of 1 orange
pink Himalayan sea salt to taste
pepper to taste
½ cup chicken broth or water (optional)

### INSTRUCTIONS

**1.** In a sealed plastic bag, marinate the whole chicken with 5 sprigs of thyme, oregano, mustard, wine, orange juice, and grated onion and refrigerate for 4 hours.

**2.** In a baking dish, make a bed with half a head of garlic, the leek, the pepper, the onion, and the celery stalk.

**3.** Place the chicken on top of the vegetable bed, spray it with olive oil, and season with the orange zest, salt, and pepper to taste. Add the juice from the marinade, and add more thyme and fresh oregano.

*(Recipe continues)*

**DAY 17**

**4.** Preheat the oven to 350°F and bake for 60 minutes. If it starts to look dry, moisten with chicken broth or water. After 60 minutes, take the tray out of the oven and turn the chicken carefully. Return it to the oven and bake for another 15 minutes or until it has reached the desired degree of doneness. Serve and enjoy.

**YIELD: 60 oz chicken and baked vegetables**

# pumpkin puree

### INGREDIENTS

1 pumpkin (15 oz)
olive oil spray
1 tbsp paprika
1 tsp five-spices seasoning
4 garlic cloves, roasted
¼ cup almond milk
pink Himalayan sea salt to taste
pepper to taste

### INSTRUCTIONS

**1.** Cut open the pumpkin, clean it well, and cut it into wedges.

**2.** Place the pumpkin pieces in a nonstick baking dish, spray them with olive oil, and season them with the paprika and the five-spices seasoning.

**3.** Bake at 350°F for 35 minutes or until cooked and soft. Remove.

**4.** Place the cooked pumpkin in the food processor along with the garlic, almond milk, salt, and pepper. Serve and enjoy.

**YIELD: 14.6 oz**

# green salad

See recipe on page 104.

| 1,200-CALORIE PLAN | 1,500-CALORIE PLAN | 1,800-CALORIE PLAN |
|---|---|---|
| ▶ 4½ oz roasted chicken + 2½ oz pumpkin puree + 1 bowl green salad | ▶ 5.3 oz roasted chicken + 5 oz pumpkin puree + 1 bowl green salad | ▶ 6½ oz roasted chicken + 7½ oz pumpkin puree + 1 bowl green salad |

DAY 17

## MEAL 4: SNACK P.M. 1:
**Almond Cinnamon Protein Greek Yogurt**

**INGREDIENTS**

1 cup Greek yogurt
½ scoop of vanilla whey protein
1 tsp cinnamon
1 stevia packet
¼ cup almonds, sliced or chopped

**INSTRUCTIONS**

**1.** In a bowl, mix yogurt, whey protein, cinnamon, and stevia with a wooden spoon.

**2.** Add the chopped almonds, serve, and enjoy.

YIELD: 9 oz

| 1,200-CALORIE PLAN | 1,500-CALORIE PLAN | 1,800-CALORIE PLAN |
|---|---|---|
| ▶3 oz | ▶4 oz | ▶5 oz |

## MEAL 5: DINNER:
**Curry Shrimp and Grilled Vegetable Kebabs**

# curry shrimp kebabs

**INGREDIENTS**

wooden skewers
16 oz shrimp, cleaned and deveined
1 onion, cut into quarters
1 red pepper, cut into cubes
1 green pepper, cut into cubes
1 yellow pepper, cut into cubes
10 cherry tomatoes
1 tbsp curry powder
1 tbsp lemongrass paste
1 tbsp ginger paste
zest of 1 lemon
pink Himalayan sea salt to taste
pepper to taste
olive oil spray

*(Recipe continues)*

DAY 17

## INSTRUCTIONS

**1.** Moisten the skewers with water before assembling the kebabs.

**2.** Assemble the kebabs in the following order: shrimp, onion, red pepper, another shrimp, green pepper, onion, yellow pepper, shrimp, and so on until you complete the desired pattern. Top each kebab off with a cherry tomato.

**3.** Season the skewers with the curry powder, lemongrass, ginger paste, lemon zest, salt, and pepper.

**4.** Fire up the grill or heat up a frying pan, and spray with olive oil. When it's hot, put the kebabs on and cook them for 2 to 3 minutes on each side. Remove and serve.

YIELD: 7 kebabs (3.6 oz each)

# grilled vegetable kebabs

See recipe on page 162.

| 1,200-CALORIE PLAN | 1,500-CALORIE PLAN | 1,800-CALORIE PLAN |
|---|---|---|
| ▶ 1½ shrimp kebabs + 1 grilled vegetable kebab | ▶ 2 shrimp kebabs + up to 2 grilled vegetable kebabs | ▶ 3 shrimp kebabs + up to 3 grilled vegetable kebabs |

## MEAL 6: SNACK P.M. 2:
### Avocado Lemon Egg Salad

### INGREDIENTS

2 hard-boiled eggs, chopped
¼ cup avocado, chopped
2 tbsps vegetarian cheese, grated
1 cup arugula or spinach
juice of 1 lemon
pink Himalayan sea salt to taste
pepper to taste

### INSTRUCTIONS

**1.** Mix the egg with the avocado and vegetarian cheese.

**2.** Serve on a bed of arugula or spinach and add lemon and salt and pepper to taste. Serve and enjoy.

YIELD: 1 serving (8 oz)

| 1,200-CALORIE PLAN | 1,500-CALORIE PLAN | 1,800-CALORIE PLAN |
|---|---|---|
| ▶ ½ cup | ▶ ½ cup | ▶ ¾ cup |

DAY 17

THE HOT BODY DIET

## Day 18

Nothing is free. Nobody is going to give you anything. No girl will bring you her boyfriend to make you happy. If you want love, admiration, and desirability, work to earn it. Don't expect to find in others what you don't have yourself. Do you want a strong and attractive man by your side? Become who you want to be, because you are the measure.

## MEAL 1: PRE-WORKOUT SNACK:
### Egg Whites + Antioxidant Smoothie

See Egg Whites recipe on page 91 and Antioxidant Smoothie recipe on page 175.

## MEAL 2: BREAKFAST:
### Vegetable Egg White Omelette + Sweet Potato Hash Browns

# vegetable egg white omelette

**INGREDIENTS**

1 egg plus 3 egg whites
¼ cup mushrooms, chopped
½ cup spinach leaves, chopped
1 tbsp red pepper, finely chopped
1 tbsp purple onion or chives, finely chopped
1 tsp sun-dried tomatoes, without oil, chopped
olive oil spray
1 tbsp almond cheese
salt to taste
pepper to taste

**INSTRUCTIONS**

**1.** Mix eggs, mushrooms, spinach, red pepper, purple onions or chives, and sun-dried tomatoes with a fork in a bowl.

*(Recipe continues)*

DAY 18

**2.** Heat a nonstick skillet, sprayed with olive oil, over medium heat, and add the egg-and-vegetable mixture. Cover it and allow it to set slightly.

**3.** Add the almond cheese and close the omelette. Add salt and pepper to taste. Serve and enjoy.

YIELD: 1 omelette

# sweet potato hash browns

### INGREDIENTS

½ cup sweet potatoes, grated (2.45 oz)
1 egg white
1 tbsp almond flour
salt to taste
pepper to taste
olive oil spray

### INSTRUCTIONS

**1.** Mix the sweet potatoes, egg white, almond flour, salt, and pepper.

**2.** Heat a nonstick skillet, sprayed with olive oil, over medium heat, and add the egg-and-potato mixture. Cover it and wait for it to cook; then flip it to the other side. Serve and enjoy.

YIELD: 1 serving (3.8 oz)

| 1,200-CALORIE PLAN | 1,500-CALORIE PLAN | 1,800-CALORIE PLAN |
|---|---|---|
| ▶ 1 omelette + ½ serving of sweet potato hash browns | ▶ 1½ omelettes + 1 serving of sweet potato hash browns | ▶ 2 omelettes + 1 serving of sweet potato hash browns |

## MEAL 3: LUNCH:
### Grilled Salmon, Arugula, and Pomegranate Salad

### INGREDIENTS

2 wild-caught salmon fillets, skinless (16 oz)
¼ cup orange juice
zest of 1 orange
1 tsp paprika powder
1 tbsp fresh dill, finely chopped
olive oil spray
1 cup fennel, finely chopped
½ cup radishes, thinly sliced

½ cup purple onion, thinly sliced
½ cup fresh pomegranate pulp
½ cup green apple, finely chopped
zest and juice of 1 lemon
1 tbsp apple cider vinegar
red pepper flakes to taste
1 cup arugula leaves, chopped

**INSTRUCTIONS**

**1.** Cut salmon fillets into cubes or strips about 1 inch wide.

**2.** In a sealed plastic bag, marinate the salmon with the orange juice, orange zest, paprika, and dill. Refrigerate for at least 1 hour.

**3.** Fire up the grill, or heat a frying pan or griddle over high heat and spray it with olive oil, and cook the salmon strips until browned on all sides. Remove and set aside.

**4.** In a large bowl, add the fennel, radish, purple onion, pomegranate, and apple, and season with the lemon zest, lemon juice, vinegar, and red pepper flakes to taste.

**5.** To serve, place the grilled salmon strips on the salad and top with the arugula and the rest of the dressing.

YIELD: 3 servings (8.6 oz each)

| 1,200-CALORIE PLAN | 1,500-CALORIE PLAN | 1,800-CALORIE PLAN |
|---|---|---|
| ▶6.6 oz | ▶8.6 oz | ▶11 oz |

## MEAL 4: SNACK P.M. 1:
### Green Apple or Pear + Peanut Butter

**INGREDIENTS**

1 green apple or pear
1 tbsp homemade peanut butter

**INSTRUCTIONS**

Wash the green apple or pear and cut it into quarters, leaving the skin. Serve with peanut butter.

YIELD: 8 oz apple or pear + 0.6 oz peanut butter

| 1,200-CALORIE PLAN | 1,500-CALORIE PLAN | 1,800-CALORIE PLAN |
|---|---|---|
| ▶½ apple or pear + 1 tbsp homemade peanut butter | ▶1 apple or pear + 1 tbsp homemade peanut butter | ▶1 apple or pear + 1 tbsp homemade peanut butter |

DAY 18

# MEAL 5: DINNER:
## Seafood and Stir-Fried Vegetable Soup

### INGREDIENTS

FOR THE STIR-FRY
olive oil spray
¼ cup onion, diced
4 garlic cloves, crushed
½ tsp ginger, grated
pinch of red pepper flakes
¼ cup chives, finely chopped
¼ cup celery, finely chopped
¼ cup sweet chili or red pepper, diced
¼ cup green pepper, diced
½ bulb fennel, diced
1 tbsp tomato, diced
pink Himalayan sea salt to taste
pepper to taste
¼ cup tomato puree

FOR THE SOUP
30 oz seafood (shrimp, scallops, squid, mussels, octopus, clams, etc.)
salt to taste
pepper to taste
1 tbsp paprika
zest of 1 large lemon
5 cups shrimp, lobster, octopus, or fish broth
¼ cup cilantro with finely chopped stems

### INSTRUCTIONS

**1.** In a heavy-bottomed pot sprayed with olive oil, place the onion, garlic, ginger, and red pepper flakes. Sauté over medium heat for two minutes.

**2.** Add the chives, celery, sweet chili or red pepper, green pepper, fennel, and tomato and mix, little by little. Add salt and pepper and cook for about 10 minutes.

**3.** Add the tomato puree to the stir-fried vegetables, and cook for 3 minutes. Remove and set aside.

**4.** Season the seafood with salt, pepper, paprika, and lemon zest.

**5.** In the same heavy-bottomed pot, sprayed with olive oil again, toss the seafood for a few minutes, until brown and crispy but still juicy.

DAY 18

THE HOT BODY DIET

**6.** Add the stir-fry and the broth and let cook for 5 minutes over medium heat. Remove from heat and add cilantro before serving.

YIELD: 40 oz

1,200-CALORIE PLAN
▶ 1¾ cups

1,500-CALORIE PLAN
▶ 2 cups

1,800-CALORIE PLAN
▶ 2½ cups

## MEAL 6: SNACK P.M. 2:
### Banana Walnut Fit Protein Cupcake

See recipe on page 89.

1,200-CALORIE PLAN
▶ ½ cupcake

1,500-CALORIE PLAN
▶ 1 cupcake

1,800-CALORIE PLAN
▶ 1 cupcake*
*You can eat a maximum of 1½ cupcakes.

DAY 18

## Day 19

Keep going! Never stop. There is nothing better than seeing the fools who criticized or rejected you when you weren't so beautiful now begging you to go out with them, offering you great opportunities, or trying to act funny for you. Pass them over and enjoy.

## MEAL 1: PRE-WORKOUT SNACK:
### Egg Whites + Antioxidant Smoothie

See Egg Whites recipe on page 91 and Antioxidant Smoothie recipe on page 175.

## MEAL 2: BREAKFAST:
### Cinnamon Protein Waffles

**INGREDIENTS**

⅓ cup rolled oats (1.2 oz)
2 egg whites
1 scoop of vanilla whey protein
⅓ cup almond milk
1 tsp cinnamon
1 packet stevia
vegetable oil spray
maple syrup (sugar-free)

**INSTRUCTIONS**

**1.** In a blender, blend oats, egg whites, whey protein, almond milk, cinnamon, and stevia for 1 minute.

**2.** Heat a waffle pan and spray it with vegetable oil. Pour half the mixture into the waffle pan and close it. Once the waffle turns golden (or the light on the waffle pan changes from red to green), remove it.

**3.** Serve with sugar-free maple syrup and enjoy!

YIELD: 2 waffles (2.3 oz each)

| 1,200-CALORIE PLAN | 1,500-CALORIE PLAN | 1,800-CALORIE PLAN |
|---|---|---|
| ► 1½ waffles | ► 2 waffles | ► 2½ waffles |

DAY 19

**THE HOT BODY DIET**

# MEAL 3: LUNCH:

## Greek Salad with Chicken and Nonfat Feta Cheese

### INGREDIENTS

**FOR THE SALAD**
6 radishes, thinly sliced
½ cup purple onion, thinly sliced
1 garlic clove, crushed
zest of 1 lemon
pink Himalayan sea salt to taste
1 tsp za'atar
1 tbsp apple cider vinegar
1 tsp paprika
10 oz chicken breast, diced
pepper to taste
1 tbsp fresh dill, chopped
olive oil spray
2 cups romaine lettuce, chopped
1 bunch of mint
1 cup red, yellow, and orange cherry tomatoes, cut into halves
1 medium cucumber, peeled, seeded, and cut into cubes
¼ cup black olives
¼ cup fat-free feta cheese, crumbled

**FOR THE VINAIGRETTE**
⅓ cup apple cider vinegar
1 tbsp extra-virgin olive oil
1 tbsp fresh dill, chopped
pink Himalayan sea salt to taste
pepper to taste

### INSTRUCTIONS

**1.** In a small bowl, place radishes and onions, with a garlic clove, lemon zest, salt, za'atar, 1 tablespoon of vinegar, and paprika. Let stand for 20 to 30 minutes.

**2.** To prepare the vinaigrette, mix the vinegar, olive oil, dill, salt, and pepper in another bowl and set aside.

**3.** Season the diced raw chicken with salt, pepper, and dill. Heat a nonstick skillet or grill, sprayed with olive oil, and add the chicken. When it's golden, remove and reserve.

*(Recipe continues)*

DAY 19

**4.** In a salad bowl, combine lettuce leaves and mint. Add the radish-and-onion mixture, chicken, chopped cherry tomatoes, cucumbers, olives, and crumbled fat-free feta cheese.

**5.** Mix everything very well.

**6.** Add the vinaigrette before serving, and enjoy.

YIELD: 3 bowls (11.3 oz each)

| 1,200-CALORIE PLAN | 1,500-CALORIE PLAN | 1,800-CALORIE PLAN |
|---|---|---|
| ▶1 bowl (11.3 oz) | ▶1½ bowls (17 oz) | ▶2 bowls (22.6 oz) |

## MEAL 4: SNACK P.M. 1:
### Turkey and Mushroom Scrambled Eggs

INGREDIENTS

1 egg plus 2 egg whites
2 slices of low-fat turkey breast ham
½ cup mushrooms, chopped
1 tbsp sun-dried tomatoes, finely chopped
olive oil spray
pinch of oregano
salt to taste
pepper to taste

INSTRUCTIONS

**1.** Mix eggs, turkey, mushrooms, and sun-dried tomatoes.

**2.** Heat a nonstick skillet, spray it with olive oil, and when it's hot, add the egg mixture.

**3.** Mix constantly with the help of a wooden spatula, and add a pinch of oregano and salt and pepper to taste.

**4.** Serve and enjoy.

YIELD: 1 serving (9 oz)

| 1,200-CALORIE PLAN | 1,500-CALORIE PLAN | 1,800-CALORIE PLAN |
|---|---|---|
| ▶4½ oz | ▶6.8 oz | ▶9 oz |

DAY 19

## MEAL 5: DINNER:

**Tuna Lettuce Wraps + Pico de Gallo**

### INGREDIENTS

10 large, clean romaine lettuce or cabbage leaves

24 oz Tuna Stew (see recipe on page 131)

6 tbsps Pico de Gallo (see recipe on page 113)

zest of 2 lemons

cilantro to taste

### INSTRUCTIONS

Use the lettuce or cabbage leaves as if they were tortillas and add the prepared Tuna Stew along with a tablespoon of Pico de Gallo. Top with lemon zest and fresh cilantro. Serve and enjoy.

**YIELD: 10 wraps (2.8 oz each)**

| 1,200-CALORIE PLAN | 1,500-CALORIE PLAN | 1,800-CALORIE PLAN |
|---|---|---|
| ►Up to 3 tuna lettuce wraps (2.8 oz each) | ►Up to 4 tuna lettuce wraps (2.8 oz each) | ►Up to 6 tuna lettuce wraps (2.8 oz each) |

## MEAL 6: SNACK P.M. 2:

**Greek Yogurt Blueberry Shake**

### INGREDIENTS

½ cup nonfat Greek yogurt

½ cup fresh blueberries

½ cup water

½ banana

juice of 1 lemon

zest of ½ lemon

stevia to taste

### INSTRUCTIONS

Process all the ingredients in a blender for 1 minute. Serve and enjoy.

**YIELD: 1 glass (8.3 oz)**

| 1,200-CALORIE PLAN | 1,500-CALORIE PLAN | 1,800-CALORIE PLAN |
|---|---|---|
| ►6 oz | ►7 oz | ►8 oz |

DAY 19

*Day 20*

There's no tomorrow. There is no later. Do it today. It is always today. One day at a time you will conquer your goal. Because if you focus on your end goal, you'll probably feel anxious. Your goal is to end each day with at least 90 percent of your goals met.

## MEAL 1: PRE-WORKOUT SNACK:
**Egg Whites + Antioxidant Smoothie**

See Egg Whites recipe on page 91 and Antioxidant Smoothie recipe on page 175.

## MEAL 2: BREAKFAST:
**Egg and Vegetable Pizza + Sweet Potato Cubes**

# egg and vegetable pizza

### INGREDIENTS

- 1 egg plus 2 egg whites
- 2 tbsps almond flour
- 1 cup raw cauliflower or broccoli, finely chopped
- 1 tsp oregano
- olive oil spray
- 2 tbsps Tomato Ragout (see recipe on page 148)
- 2 turkey breasts, thinly sliced
- ½ cup mushrooms
- 2 tbsps vegetarian mozzarella cheese

### INSTRUCTIONS

**1.** In a food processor, mix the eggs, almond flour, cauliflower or broccoli, and oregano until you obtain a smooth mixture.

**2.** Heat a nonstick skillet over medium heat, spray it with olive oil, and add the egg mixture. Cover and wait until the mixture is cooked, making sure it browns on the bottom.

**3.** Add the Tomato Ragout, turkey breast slices, and mushrooms and top it off with the vegetarian cheese. Cover again until the cheese melts. (You can also do this last step in the oven.)

**4.** Serve and enjoy.

YIELD: 6.05 oz

## sweet potato cubes

**INGREDIENTS**

35 oz sweet potatoes or yams
olive oil spray
cinnamon, cumin, thyme, or oregano for flavor
salt to taste
pepper to taste

**INSTRUCTIONS**

**1.** Wash and dry the sweet potatoes, leaving the skin on, and cut them lengthwise and then transversely several times to make cubes.

**2.** Spray them with olive oil and season with the seasoning of your preference, and salt and pepper to taste.

**3.** Bake in a baking dish at 350°F for 25 to 30 minutes until golden brown.

YIELD: 20 oz

**1,200-CALORIE PLAN**
▶ ⅓ pizza (2 oz) + 1¼ oz sweet potato cubes

**1,500-CALORIE PLAN**
▶ ⅓ pizza (2 oz) + 2½ oz sweet potato cubes

**1,800-CALORIE PLAN**
▶ ⅔ pizza (4 oz) + 2½ oz sweet potato cubes

DAY 20

# grilled steak

**INGREDIENTS**

1 tbsp BBQ seasoning
1 tsp paprika
1 tsp chili powder
pink Himalayan sea salt to taste
16 oz beef tenderloin, clean
olive oil spray

**INSTRUCTIONS**

**1.** In a small bowl, mix the BBQ seasoning, paprika, chili powder, and salt.

**2.** Spray the whole piece of meat with olive oil and rub it with spices and salt, making sure to cover every part.

**3.** Fire up the grill or heat the griddle on high heat and place the piece of meat on it to roast; it should become brown on all sides. When it reaches the desired degree of doneness, remove it from the heat and let it stand before serving.

YIELD: 13.3 oz

# grilled vegetables

**INGREDIENTS**

1 zucchini
1 eggplant
1 red pepper
1 yellow pepper
1 artichoke heart
1 portobello mushroom
olive oil spray
Italian herbs (rosemary, sage, oregano, thyme, and basil)
pink Himalayan sea salt to taste
pepper to taste

**INSTRUCTIONS**

**1.** Cut the zucchini and eggplant into slices ¼ inch thick. Quarter the peppers, the artichoke heart, and the portobello mushroom.

**2.** Heat a grill or griddle to high heat, spray it with olive oil, and season the vegetables with the Italian herbs, pink Himalayan sea salt, and pepper. Place them on the grill or griddle for 2 minutes on each side and remove.

YIELD: 28.3 oz

## *guasacaca*

### INGREDIENTS

2 ripe avocados crushed with a fork
1 red onion, diced
1 tomato, seedless, diced
½ red pepper, diced
2 hot chilies, finely diced
1 garlic clove, minced
juice of 1 lemon
1 tbsp apple cider vinegar
pink Himalayan sea salt to taste
pepper to taste
1 bunch cilantro, finely chopped, to taste (optional)
zest of 1 lemon (optional)

### INSTRUCTIONS

Mix all ingredients, including the fresh cilantro and lemon zest (if desired). Adjust the seasoning and place in a serving bowl.

YIELD: 19.6 oz

| 1,200-CALORIE PLAN | 1,500-CALORIE PLAN | 1,800-CALORIE PLAN |
|---|---|---|
| ▶ 4 oz grilled steak + 9 oz grilled vegetables + 2.3 oz *guasacaca* | ▶ 5 oz grilled steak + 9 oz grilled vegetables + 3½ oz *guasacaca* | ▶ 7 oz grilled steak + 9 oz grilled vegetables + 4.6 oz *guasacaca* |

## MEAL 4: SNACK P.M. 1:
### Walnut Raisin Fit Protein Cupcake

See recipe on page 89.

| 1,200-CALORIE PLAN | 1,500-CALORIE PLAN | 1,800-CALORIE PLAN |
|---|---|---|
| ▶ ½ cupcake | ▶ 1 cupcake | ▶ 1 cupcake*<br>*You can eat a maximum of 1½ cupcakes. |

DAY 20

# MEAL 5: DINNER:
## Fish and Vegetable Soup

### INGREDIENTS

16 oz whitefish fillet (corvina, sea bass, or tilapia), cut in cubes
1 tsp paprika
1 tsp garlic, crushed
zest of 1 lemon
olive oil spray
water
½ cup onion, julienned
½ cup leeks, julienned
½ cup fennel, julienned
½ cup carrots, julienned
½ cup green beans, chopped
4 cups fish or vegetable broth
1 tbsp sriracha sauce
pink Himalayan sea salt to taste
cilantro to taste
fresh chives to taste

### INSTRUCTIONS

**1.** Season the fish cubes with paprika, garlic, and lemon zest.

**2.** Heat a heavy-bottomed pot over high heat, spray it with olive oil, and cook the fish cubes. When the fish is sufficiently golden but still juicy, add a little water to deglaze the cooking juices. Remove the fish and reserve.

**3.** In the same pot, spray olive oil and gradually add the onions, leeks, fennel, carrots, and green beans. Stir-fry for a few minutes, until the vegetables soften.

**4.** Add the broth and the fish, then the sriracha, salt, cilantro, and chives.

**5.** Adjust the seasoning, serve, and enjoy.

**YIELD: 40 oz**

| 1,200-CALORIE PLAN | 1,500-CALORIE PLAN | 1,800-CALORIE PLAN |
|---|---|---|
| ▶ 1¼ cups soup | ▶ 1½ cups soup | ▶ 2 cups soup |

**DAY 20**

**THE HOT BODY DIET**

## MEAL 6: SNACK P.M. 2:

**Tuna Stew**

See recipe on page 131.

| 1,200-CALORIE PLAN | 1,500-CALORIE PLAN | 1,800-CALORIE PLAN |
|---|---|---|
| ▶4 oz | ▶6 oz | ▶8 oz |

# Day 21

You are already on your twenty-first day. And if you haven't yet failed, let me tell you that you've reached the point of no return! Congratulations! You made it. Keep going: the results are much closer than they were, and your spirit is already very strong. From now on, you will be unstoppable.

## MEAL 1: PRE-WORKOUT SNACK:
**Egg Whites + Antioxidant Smoothie**

See Egg Whites recipe on page 91 and Antioxidant Smoothie recipe on page 175.

## MEAL 2: BREAKFAST:
**Chia Protein Pancakes**

**INGREDIENTS**

⅓ cup rolled oats
1 egg plus 2 egg whites
½ scoop of chocolate whey protein
1 tsp unsweetened cocoa powder
1 tsp chia seeds and flaxseeds
1 tsp stevia
½ tsp vanilla
½ tsp baking powder
2 tbsps almond milk or water
vegetable oil spray

**INSTRUCTIONS**

**1.** Mix all ingredients except the vegetable oil spray in a blender.

**2.** Heat a nonstick skillet over medium heat, spray it with vegetable oil, and add a third of the mixture.

**3.** Cover it, wait for it to brown a little, and flip it immediately to cook on the other side.

YIELD: 3 pancakes (2.1 oz each)

| 1,200-CALORIE PLAN | 1,500-CALORIE PLAN | 1,800-CALORIE PLAN |
|---|---|---|
| ▶ 1 pancake | ▶ 2 pancakes | ▶ 3 pancakes |

# lemon grilled fish

### INGREDIENTS

   16 oz whitefish fillet (sea bass, snapper, grouper, catfish, barracuda,
      tilapia, corvina, saw, sole, anchovy, etc.)
   1 garlic clove, grated
   zest of 1 lemon
   pink Himalayan sea salt to taste
   pepper to taste
   olive oil spray
   juice of 1 lemon

### INSTRUCTIONS

**1.** In a bowl, season the fish fillets, cut into 3-inch strips, with grated garlic, lemon zest, salt, and pepper.

**2.** Heat a nonstick skillet, grill, or griddle to high heat and spray it with olive oil. Spray fish fillets with oil, place them on the skillet, grill, or griddle, and turn them carefully when golden, to sear them on both sides.

**3.** Add the lemon juice to deglaze the sauce, and serve immediately.

**YIELD: 12.6 oz**

# sweet potato puree

See recipe on page 93.

# pineapple coleslaw salad

See recipe on page 168.

| 1,200-CALORIE PLAN | 1,500-CALORIE PLAN | 1,800-CALORIE PLAN |
|---|---|---|
| ► 5.8 oz fish + 2 oz sweet potato puree + 1 cup pineapple coleslaw salad | ► 7 oz fish + 4 oz sweet potato puree + 1 cup pineapple coleslaw salad | ► 10 oz fish + 6 oz sweet potato puree + 1 cup pineapple coleslaw salad |

**DAY 21**

## MEAL 4: SNACK P.M. 1:

**Unsalted Nuts**

Choose a serving of almonds, cashews, pistachios, or peanuts.

**1,200-CALORIE PLAN**
- Almonds or cashews: 0.8 oz or up to 12 nuts
- Pistachios: ½ oz or up to 25 nuts
- Peanuts (unsalted): ½ oz or up to 20 nuts

**1,500-CALORIE PLAN**
- Almonds or cashews: 1.3 oz or up to 18 nuts
- Pistachios: 0.8 oz or up to 40 nuts
- Peanuts (unsalted): 0.7 oz or up to 30 nuts

**1,800-CALORIE PLAN**
- Almonds or cashews: 1.6 oz or up to 24 nuts
- Pistachios: 1 oz or up to 50 nuts
- Peanuts (unsalted): 0.9 oz or up to 40 nuts

Or, if you want to eat a combination, these are the suggested serving sizes:

**1,200-CALORIE PLAN**
- 4 almonds or cashews + 9 pistachios + 6 peanuts (unsalted)

**1,500-CALORIE PLAN**
- 6 almonds or cashews + 14 pistachios + 10 peanuts (unsalted)

**1,800-CALORIE PLAN**
- 8 almonds or cashews + 18 pistachios + 13 peanuts (unsalted)

## MEAL 5: DINNER:

**Cheat Meal**

## MEAL 6: SNACK P.M. 2:

**Light Pineapple Gelatin (optional)**

### INGREDIENTS

- 1 cup hot water
- 1 cup almond milk without sugar (cold)
- 1 box of pineapple- or orange-flavored gelatin, sugar-free
- 1 small pineapple, chopped into small pieces

### INSTRUCTIONS

**1.** Heat 1 cup of water.

**2.** In a large bowl, mix 1 cup of hot water with the almond milk and then add the contents of the gelatin box as well as the chopped pineapple.

DAY 21

**3.** Refrigerate until cool and firm. Serve and enjoy.

**YIELD: 4 cups (8 oz each)**

| 1,200-CALORIE PLAN | 1,500-CALORIE PLAN | 1,800-CALORIE PLAN |
|---|---|---|
| ▶Up to 2 cups | ▶Up to 4 cups | ▶Up to 6 cups |

## SUPERSTAR RECIPE OF THE WEEK

# bison and pumpkin burger

**INGREDIENTS**

- 4 oz ground bison, turkey, or chicken
- 2 tbsps almond flour
- salt to taste
- garlic powder to taste
- pepper to taste
- olive oil spray
- 4 oz Pumpkin Puree (see recipe on page 188) or Baked Sweet Potato (see recipe on page 103)
- 3 tbsps oat bran
- 1 egg white
- 1 tsp chia seeds
- 1 tsp flaxseeds
- arugula, alfalfa, or spinach to taste
- 2 slices of tomato
- mustard to taste

**INSTRUCTIONS**

**1.** In a bowl, mix the ground meat with the almond flour, salt, garlic powder, and pepper to taste.

**2.** To prepare the burger, take the meat mixture and form it into a ball about the size of your palm.

**3.** Heat a nonstick skillet sprayed with olive oil over medium heat and cook the hamburger until golden brown. Flip and repeat the procedure. Set aside.

**4.** Use a food processor or spatula and a separate bowl to mash the pumpkin with the oat bran and egg white. Add the chia seeds, flaxseeds, and more salt and pepper to taste.

**5.** To prepare the pumpkin tops, take half of the mixture and form it into palm-sized balls. Then do the same with the other half.

**6.** Heat the pumpkin tops in a nonstick pan sprayed with olive oil over medium heat. Cook until golden brown. Then flip them and repeat the procedure. Set aside and let cool.

**7.** Serve the burger on a flat plate, placing it on a pumpkin lid and topping with arugula, alfalfa, or spinach, tomato, and mustard. Cover at the end with another pumpkin top and enjoy!

**YIELD: 1 burger (10 oz)**

You can switch this recipe up in many ways. You can substitute bison meat with chicken, turkey, or ground fish prepared as burger patties. You can also swap the pumpkin with sweet potatoes, yucca, or green bananas.

## Day 22

There is no dessert more satisfying than seeing yourself in the mirror and finding a fit and healthy body. Look at yourself in the mirror and enjoy the changes that are starting to emerge. Feel the happiness of walking around in pants that aren't tight. Above all, feel proud of how strong you are today.

## MEAL 1: PRE-WORKOUT SNACK:
**Egg Whites + Pineapple Skin Infusion**

See Egg Whites recipe on page 91.

## pineapple skin infusion

**INGREDIENTS**

8 cups of water
skin of 1 pineapple
4 pineapple slices, chopped
4 cinnamon sticks
10 whole cloves
lemon to taste
stevia to taste

**INSTRUCTIONS**

1. Bring 8 cups of water to a boil.
2. Add the fresh pineapple skin, the chopped pineapple, the cinnamon, and the cloves.
3. Allow the liquid to boil and reduce by at least half.
4. Strain to remove pineapple skin, cinnamon, and cloves.
5. Serve hot or cold with lemon and stevia to taste.

YIELD: 8 cups

| 1,200-CALORIE PLAN | 1,500-CALORIE PLAN | 1,800-CALORIE PLAN |
|---|---|---|
| ▶8 oz | ▶12 oz | ▶16 oz |

# MEAL 2: BREAKFAST:
## Baked Eggs in Stuffed Peppers

### INGREDIENTS

1 red pepper
2 eggs plus 2 egg whites
2 tsps almond cheese
parsley or cilantro, finely chopped
pink Himalayan sea salt to taste
pepper to taste

### INSTRUCTIONS

**1.** Take a red pepper and cut it in half lengthwise, removing all seeds.

**2.** Fill each half of the pepper with 1 egg and 1 egg white.

**3.** Sprinkle the grated almond cheese over the two halves and bake at 350°F for 25 minutes.

**4.** Remove from the oven and add fresh parsley or cilantro, salt, and pepper.

**5.** Serve and enjoy.

YIELD: 1 serving (12 oz)

| 1,200-CALORIE PLAN | 1,500-CALORIE PLAN | 1,800-CALORIE PLAN |
|---|---|---|
| ►9 oz | ►12 oz | ►18 oz |

DAY 22

## MEAL 3: LUNCH:
### Thai Chicken Vegetable Stir-Fry

**INGREDIENTS**

FOR THE MARINADE

1 tbsp curry paste
½ tbsp lemongrass paste
1 tbsp ginger, grated
½ tbsp sriracha sauce
¼ tsp five-spices seasoning
½ cup water
1 tbsp rice vinegar
1 tbsp natural tamarind paste, without seeds
2 stevia packets

FOR THE STIR-FRY

16 oz chicken breast, diced
olive oil spray
½ cup onion, cut into large wedges
½ cup red and yellow peppers cut into large wedges
½ cup mushrooms, diced
½ cup broccoli, chopped
½ cup bean or lentil sprouts
2 tbsps chives, finely chopped
1 tbsp unsalted peanuts
2 tbsps spring onions, finely chopped

**INSTRUCTIONS**

**1.** To prepare the marinade, place all the ingredients in a blender and process until you obtain a smooth mixture. Set aside.

**2.** Place the diced chicken breast and the marinade in a sealed plastic bag, and keep refrigerated for 4 to 8 hours.

**3.** Place a large pan or wok over high heat and spray it with olive oil. Immediately add the marinated chicken and cook until brown. Remove the chicken from the pan and set it aside.

**4.** Take the same pan, spray it again with olive oil, and sauté the vegetables by adding them in the following order: onions, peppers, mushrooms, and broccoli, and at the very end, add the sprouts and the chives. The vegetables should be cooked but crunchy.

DAY 22

**5.** Add the marinated chicken and toss everything together until the flavors are nicely blended. Remove from the heat and sprinkle with peanuts and spring onions before serving.

YIELD: 26.3 oz

| 1,200-CALORIE PLAN | 1,500-CALORIE PLAN | 1,800-CALORIE PLAN |
|---|---|---|
| ▶ 5.6 oz | ▶ 6½ oz | ▶ 10 oz |

## MEAL 4: SNACK P.M. 1:
### Artichoke and Spinach Hummus + Carrot Sticks

**INGREDIENTS**

1 cup natural chickpeas
pink Himalayan sea salt to taste
juice of 2 or 3 medium lemons
¼ cup tahini or sesame cream
1 tbsp olive oil
2 large garlic cloves, crushed
2 cooked artichoke hearts
½ cup spinach, raw
1 large carrot, cut into sticks

**INSTRUCTIONS**

**1.** Cook the chickpeas in 1 quart of water with Himalayan sea salt until they are soft. Drain well.

**2.** Transfer the chickpeas to a food processor, along with lemon juice, tahini or sesame cream, olive oil, salt to taste, and crushed garlic.

**3.** Add the artichoke hearts and the raw spinach and process until you obtain a homogenous paste.

**4.** Serve with carrot sticks.

YIELD: 1½ cups hummus (12 oz)

| 1,200-CALORIE PLAN | 1,500-CALORIE PLAN | 1,800-CALORIE PLAN |
|---|---|---|
| ▶ 3 oz hummus + 4 carrot sticks | ▶ Up to 5 oz hummus + 6 carrot sticks | ▶ Up to 7 oz hummus + 6 carrot sticks |

DAY 22

## MEAL 5: DINNER:
**Asian Chicken Salad + Asian Vinaigrette**

See recipe on page 118.


## MEAL 6: SNACK P.M. 2:
**Strawberry Protein Pancakes**

See recipe on page 111.

DAY 22

## Day 23

The best thing about changing your lifestyle is that you will gain joy, self-esteem, strength, enthusiasm, and energy; that's even more important than your physical transformation. You will begin to shine with such a bright light that you will blind anyone who tries to look at you. You will never go unnoticed.

## MEAL 1: PRE-WORKOUT SNACK:
### Egg Whites + Pineapple Skin Infusion

See Egg Whites recipe on page 91 and Pineapple Skin Infusion recipe on page 212.

## MEAL 2: BREAKFAST:
### Bison and Pumpkin Burger

See recipe on page 210.

| 1,200-CALORIE PLAN | 1,500-CALORIE PLAN | 1,800-CALORIE PLAN |
|---|---|---|
| ▶ ½ burger (5 oz) | ▶ ¾ burger (7½ oz) | ▶ 1 burger (10 oz) |

DAY 23

# fish in sesame sauce

### INGREDIENTS

16 oz whitefish fillets (sea bass, corvina, snapper, grouper, tilapia, dorado, or barracuda)

pink Himalayan sea salt to taste

pepper to taste

2½ tbsps tahini

2 tbsps lemon juice

2 tbsps lemon zest

2 garlic cloves, crushed

2 tbsps water

olive oil spray

1 large white onion, julienned

½ cup parsley, finely chopped

### INSTRUCTIONS

**1.** Season the fish with salt and pepper.

**2.** To prepare the sesame sauce, place the tahini, lemon juice, lemon zest, crushed garlic, and water in a blender and blend until you obtain a creamy sauce. Set aside.

**3.** Spray a well-heated skillet with olive oil and add the fish to sear it on both sides. Set aside.

**4.** Spray the same pan with a little olive oil and sauté the onion until it turns golden but without letting it burn.

**5.** Preheat the oven to 375°F. Transfer the fish and the sautéed onions to a baking dish and cover with the sesame sauce.

**6.** Bake for 15 to 20 minutes and remove from the oven. Sprinkle with chopped parsley and serve.

YIELD: 18 oz

# *fattoush* salad

### INGREDIENTS

#### FOR THE DRESSING

1 tbsp olive oil

1 tsp sumac

DAY 23

1 tsp za'atar

½ tsp cumin

¼ cup lemon juice

zest of 1 lemon

pink Himalayan sea salt to taste

pepper to taste

FOR THE SALAD

2 cups romaine lettuce, chopped

1 seedless cucumber, diced

1 seedless tomato, diced

¼ cup chives, finely chopped

¼ cup fresh mint leaves, chopped

1 cup fresh parsley, chopped

2 slices whole wheat toast, diced to make croutons (optional)

## INSTRUCTIONS

**1.** Prepare the dressing by whisking together all ingredients in a bowl. Set aside.

**2.** In a large bowl or on a large platter, toss together the lettuce, cucumber, tomatoes, chives, mint, and parsley, then season with the dressing.

**3.** If desired, you can top off the salad with whole wheat croutons.

**4.** Serve and enjoy.

**YIELD: 5 cups of salad and ½ cup dressing**

| 1,200-CALORIE PLAN | 1,500-CALORIE PLAN | 1,800-CALORIE PLAN |
|---|---|---|
| ▶ 6 oz fish with sesame sauce + 1 cup *fattoush* + 1 slice of whole wheat toast | ▶ 7.6 oz fish with sesame sauce + 1½ cups *fattoush* + 2 slices of whole wheat toast | ▶ 10.6 oz fish with sesame sauce + 2 cups *fattoush* + 3 slices of whole wheat toast |

## MEAL 4: SNACK P.M. 1:
### Apple Cinnamon Fit Protein Cupcake

See recipe on page 89.

| 1,200-CALORIE PLAN | 1,500-CALORIE PLAN | 1,800-CALORIE PLAN |
|---|---|---|
| ▶ ½ cupcake | ▶ 1 cupcake | ▶ 1 cupcake* *You can eat a maximum of 1½ cupcakes. |

# chicken chili lettuce wraps

**INGREDIENTS**

10 large, clean romaine lettuce or cabbage leaves
24 oz Chicken Chili (see recipe on page 134)
⅔ cup Pico de Gallo (see recipe on page 113)
fresh cilantro to taste
zest of 1 lemon

**INSTRUCTIONS**

**1.** Use the lettuce or cabbage leaves as if they were tortillas and fill them with the Chicken Chili.

**2.** Top with 1 tablespoon of Pico de Gallo, the fresh cilantro, and the lemon zest.

**YIELD: 10 wraps (2.8 oz each)**

| 1,200-CALORIE PLAN | 1,500-CALORIE PLAN | 1,800-CALORIE PLAN |
|---|---|---|
| ▶ Up to 3 lettuce wraps (2.8 oz each) | ▶ Up to 4 lettuce wraps (2.8 oz each) | ▶ Up to 6 lettuce wraps (2.8 oz each) |

## MEAL 6: SNACK P.M. 2:
### Green Apple-Smoked Salmon Rolls

**INGREDIENTS**

zest of 1 lemon
juice of ½ lemon
1 tsp fresh ginger, grated
1 tbsp light soy sauce
pepper to taste
2 slices of smoked salmon (1½ oz)
½ apple, julienned
½ cup arugula

**INSTRUCTIONS**

**1.** Prepare the dressing by mixing the lemon zest, lemon juice, ginger, soy sauce, and pepper.

**DAY 23**

**2.** Take a slice of smoked salmon and place some of the julienned green apple and the arugula on top. Roll carefully.

**3.** Serve with dressing and enjoy.

YIELD: 2 rolls

**1,200-CALORIE PLAN**
▶ 1 roll

**1,500-CALORIE PLAN**
▶ 1½ rolls

**1,800-CALORIE PLAN**
▶ 2 rolls

DAY 23

## Day 24

Do you look much better? Do you feel your muscles getting stronger? If your answer is yes, congratulations! Because you're the one responsible for that change. Conquer your mind and your body; the treasure of self-confidence will bring great things into your life. If you want your world to change, start with yourself. You will attract great things.

## MEAL 1: PRE-WORKOUT SNACK:
**Egg Whites + Pineapple Skin Infusion**

See Egg Whites recipe on page 91 and Pineapple Skin Infusion recipe on page 212.

## MEAL 2: BREAKFAST:
**Spinach and Vegetarian Cheese Omelette with Whole Wheat Toast**

# spinach and vegetarian cheese omelette with whole wheat toast

**INGREDIENTS**

1 egg plus 2 egg whites
1 tbsp leeks, finely chopped
½ cup spinach leaves
olive oil spray
2 tbsps almond cheese topping
salt to taste
pepper to taste
2 slices of whole wheat toast (high fiber, sugar-free)

**INSTRUCTIONS**

**1.** In a bowl, mix eggs, leeks, and spinach.

**2.** Place a nonstick pan on medium heat and spray it with olive oil. Add the egg mixture and allow it to cook for 1 minute.

**3.** Put the almond cheese in the middle of the omelette. Fold it and cover the pan until the omelette is thoroughly cooked. Add salt and pepper to taste.

**4.** Serve with toast and enjoy.

YIELD: 1 omelette (5.6 oz)

| 1,200-CALORIE PLAN | 1,500-CALORIE PLAN | 1,800-CALORIE PLAN |
|---|---|---|
| ▶ 1 omelette + 2 slices of high-fiber whole wheat toast | ▶ 1½ omelettes + 3 slices of high-fiber whole wheat toast | ▶ 2 omelettes + 4 slices of high-fiber whole wheat toast |

## MEAL 3: LUNCH:
### Grilled Sirloin Steak + Mixed Salad with Avocado

# grilled sirloin steak

**INGREDIENTS**

¼ tsp mustard seeds
¼ tsp peppercorns (black, pink, and green)
1 tsp garlic, crushed
Italian herbs (rosemary, sage, oregano, thyme, and basil)
pink Himalayan sea salt to taste
¼ cup red wine
16 oz beef sirloin steak
olive oil spray

**INSTRUCTIONS**

**1.** In a stone mortar or *molcajete*, grind the mustard seeds, peppercorns, garlic, herbs, and salt until you obtain a thick paste, and then add the wine. Reserve.

**2.** Place the sirloin steak on a flat surface and rub it on all sides with the paste.

**3.** On a grill or in a frying pan sprayed with olive oil, cook the steak for 5 to 7 minutes on each side over high heat until you reach the desired degree of doneness.

**4.** Remove from the heat and let sit for 5 to 8 minutes. Slice and serve.

YIELD: 15 oz

DAY 24

# mixed salad with avocado

**INGREDIENTS**

1 cup mixed greens (lettuce, romaine lettuce, purple cabbage, arugula, watercress, baby spinach, and endive)

1 tomato, diced

¼ onion, julienned

½ small avocado, diced (3½ oz)

cilantro to taste

juice of 1 lemon

1 tsp olive oil

salt to taste

pepper to taste

**INSTRUCTIONS**

1. Mix all ingredients.
2. Serve.

YIELD: 2½ bowls of salad (6 oz each)

| 1,200-CALORIE PLAN | 1,500-CALORIE PLAN | 1,800-CALORIE PLAN |
|---|---|---|
| ▶ 4 oz grilled sirloin steak + 1 bowl mixed salad with avocado | ▶ 5 oz grilled sirloin steak + 1 bowl mixed salad with avocado | ▶ 7 oz grilled sirloin steak + 1 bowl mixed salad with avocado |

## MEAL 4: SNACK P.M. 1:

### Popcorn with Turmeric and Pepper

**INGREDIENTS**

5 tbsps popcorn kernels

5 tbsps water

1 tsp turmeric powder

salt to taste

pepper to taste

**INSTRUCTIONS**

1. Place the popcorn kernels in a large, round microwave-safe container.
2. Add the water and turmeric, and the salt and pepper to taste.

DAY 24

**3.** Cover the container with plastic film, making sure it's perfectly sealed around the edges. Then with a sharp knife pierce the film 4 or 5 times.

**4.** Microwave for 5 minutes. Remove the plastic film, serve, and enjoy! The container gets very hot, so be careful when you remove it from the microwave!

YIELD: 3 cups (1.8 oz each)

| 1,200-CALORIE PLAN | 1,500-CALORIE PLAN | 1,800-CALORIE PLAN |
|---|---|---|
| ►1 cup | ►2 cups | ►3 cups |

## MEAL 5: DINNER:
Steamed Fish with Ginger + Grilled Asparagus

## steamed fish with ginger

For this dish you will need a steamer (bamboo, electric, or aluminum). If you don't have a steamer, you can prepare the meal over low heat on the grill or in the oven at 325°F.

### INGREDIENTS

16 oz fish fillet of your preference
¼ cup fresh ginger, finely chopped
¼ cup chives, finely chopped
¼ cup leeks, julienned
¼ cup carrots, finely chopped
1 tsp light soy sauce, low sodium
½ tsp sesame oil

### INSTRUCTIONS

**1.** Take a deep pot and add water up to the middle. Bring the water to a boil and place the steamer inside the pot.

**2.** Place the fish inside the steamer and cover it with the ginger, chives, leeks, and carrots. Season with soy sauce and sesame oil.

**3.** Cover and cook for 10 to 12 minutes. Serve and enjoy.

YIELD: 15 oz fish and steamed vegetables

DAY 24

# grilled asparagus

See recipe on page 117.

**1,200-CALORIE PLAN**
► 5.8 oz steamed fish + 4 oz asparagus

**1,500-CALORIE PLAN**
► 7 oz steamed fish + 6 oz asparagus

**1,800-CALORIE PLAN**
► 10 oz steamed fish + 10 oz asparagus

## MEAL 6: SNACK P.M. 2:
**Carrot Fit Protein Cupcake**

See recipe on page 89.

**1,200-CALORIE PLAN**
► ½ cupcake

**1,500-CALORIE PLAN**
► 1 cupcake

**1,800-CALORIE PLAN**
► 1 cupcake*
*You can eat a maximum of 1½ cupcakes.

## Day 25

Every triumph must be celebrated. Cheer up and love yourself! Every time you go to the gym and complete your routine you're getting stronger and more beautiful. A step at a time brings you closer to your goal. Every day is important. Every day counts.

## MEAL 1: PRE-WORKOUT SNACK:
### Egg Whites + Pineapple Skin Infusion

See Egg Whites recipe on page 91 and Pineapple Skin Infusion recipe on page 212.

## MEAL 2: BREAKFAST:
### Chocolate Chip Fit Protein Waffles

**INGREDIENTS**

⅓ cup rolled oats
2 egg whites
1 scoop of chocolate whey protein
⅓ cup almond milk
½ tsp vanilla
1 stevia packet
2 tbsps chocolate chips (sugar-free)
vegetable oil spray
maple syrup (sugar-free)

**INSTRUCTIONS**

**1.** Add the oats, egg whites, whey protein, almond milk, vanilla, and stevia to a blender and blend for 1 minute. Add the chocolate chips.

**2.** Heat a waffle pan and spray it with vegetable oil. Pour half the mixture into the waffle pan and close it. Once the waffle turns golden (or the light on the waffle pan changes from red to green), remove it.

**3.** Serve with the sugar-free maple syrup and enjoy!

YIELD: 2 waffles (2.3 oz each)

| 1,200-CALORIE PLAN | 1,500-CALORIE PLAN | 1,800-CALORIE PLAN |
|---|---|---|
| ▶ 1½ waffles | ▶ 2 waffles | ▶ 2½ waffles |

# MEAL 3: LUNCH:
## Vegetarian Cheese, Tomato, and Arugula Cauliflower Pizza

### INGREDIENTS

1 large cauliflower head

1 egg

16 oz almond vegetarian cheese, grated

pink Himalayan sea salt to taste

pepper to taste

Italian herbs (oregano, rosemary, thyme, sage, and bay leaves) to taste (optional)

1 cup Tomato Ragout (see recipe on page 148)

½ cup cherry tomatoes, chopped

¼ cup green pepper, julienned

1 cup mushrooms, sliced

½ cup arugula

1 tbsp olive oil

### INSTRUCTIONS

**1.** Clean the cauliflower, separate the florets from the stem, and transfer the florets into a high-speed food processor. Process the cauliflower in 1-second pulses until it's completely broken down.

**2.** Transfer the processed cauliflower into a bowl and cover with waxed paper. Microwave for 8 minutes.

**3.** Remove the cauliflower from the microwave and mix with the egg and half the vegetarian cheese, and season with salt, pepper, and the Italian herbs to your liking.

**4.** Transfer the cauliflower mixture onto a nonstick pan and use a spatula to flatten it and give it the shape of a pizza.

**5.** Bake the dough for 10 to 15 minutes at 325°F. Remove from the oven.

**6.** Arrange as a traditional pizza and add the Tomato Ragout, the remaining cheese, the cherry tomatoes, the green pepper, and the mushrooms.

**7.** Bake again until the cheese melts and the edges of the crust turn brown. Take the pizza out of the oven and top with the arugula, olive oil, and pepper.

**8.** Serve and enjoy.

YIELD: 28 oz

| 1,200-CALORIE PLAN | 1,500-CALORIE PLAN | 1,800-CALORIE PLAN |
|---|---|---|
| ▶ 11.6 oz | ▶ 14.2 oz | ▶ 18 oz |

DAY 25

## MEAL 4: SNACK P.M. 1:

**Blackberry Protein Ice Cream**

### INGREDIENTS

1 cup frozen blackberries (or any other berries)
1 scoop of vanilla whey protein
½ cup almond milk
zest of ½ lemon
2 stevia packets

### INSTRUCTIONS

**1.** Place the blackberries, whey protein, almond milk, lemon zest, and stevia in a food processor.

**2.** Process until you obtain a smooth and creamy mixture. Tranfer to a container and freeze until it reaches the consistency of ice cream.

**YIELD: 1½ cups (11.7 oz)**

| 1,200-CALORIE PLAN | 1,500-CALORIE PLAN | 1,800-CALORIE PLAN |
|---|---|---|
| ▶ ¾ cup (5.8 oz) | ▶ 1 cup (8 oz) | ▶ 1½ cups (11.7 oz) |

DAY 25

## MEAL 5: DINNER:
**Chicken Vegetable Stir-Fry**

**INGREDIENTS**

FOR THE MARINADE
1 tbsp grated ginger
½ tbsp sriracha sauce
½ cup orange juice
zest of 1 orange

FOR THE STIR-FRY
16 oz chicken breast, cut into 1-inch cubes
olive oil spray
½ cup onion, cut into cubes
½ cup yellow pepper, cut into cubes
½ cup red pepper, cut into cubes
1 cup mushrooms, diced
½ cup broccoli florets
½ cup zucchini, cut in half rounds
½ cup green beans
½ cup soybean sprouts
¼ cup chives, finely chopped plus more for garnish
pink Himalayan sea salt to taste
pepper to taste
1 tbsp sesame seeds, toasted

**INSTRUCTIONS**

**1.** To prepare the marinade, place all the ingredients in a blender and process until you obtain a smooth mixture. Set aside.

**2.** Transfer the marinade and the chicken cubes to a sealed bag and refrigerate for at least 4 hours. Drain.

**3.** Place a large pan or wok over high heat and spray it with olive oil. Immediately add the marinated chicken and cook until brown. Remove it from the pan and set it aside.

**4.** Take the same pan, spray it again with olive oil, and sauté the vegetables by adding them in the following order: onions, peppers, mushrooms, broccoli, zucchini, and green beans, and at the very end, add the sprouts and the chives. The vegetables should be cooked but crunchy.

DAY 25

**THE HOT BODY DIET**

**5.** Add the marinated chicken and toss everything together until the flavors are nicely blended. Remove from the heat and sprinkle with salt, pepper, sesame seeds, and chives before serving.

YIELD: 29.6 oz

| 1,200-CALORIE PLAN | 1,500-CALORIE PLAN | 1,800-CALORIE PLAN |
|---|---|---|
| ►6 oz | ►7 oz | ►10 oz |

## MEAL 6: SNACK P.M. 2:
### Turkey Breast Zucchini Rolls

**INGREDIENTS**

½ zucchini
olive oil spray
4 slices of turkey breast ham (low sodium)
alfalfa sprouts to taste
mustard to taste
¼ cup cherry tomatoes, chopped

**INSTRUCTIONS**

**1.** Using a mandoline or a sharp knife, cut the zucchini lengthwise into thin slices.

**2.** Fire up the grill or heat a pan over high heat, spray it with olive oil, and quickly sear the zucchini slices on both sides.

**3.** Arrange the rolls by filling each zucchini slice with a slice of turkey breast ham, some alfalfa sprouts, some mustard, and cherry tomatoes. Roll up carefully.

**4.** Serve and enjoy.

YIELD: 4 rolls (2.2 oz each)

| 1,200-CALORIE PLAN | 1,500-CALORIE PLAN | 1,800-CALORIE PLAN |
|---|---|---|
| ►2 rolls | ►3 rolls | ►4 rolls |

DAY 25

## Day 26

Do it again; do it better. You already know the drill. Don't lose to the refrigerator when you have gained so much at the gym. There is no bigger prize than looking good and feeling good about yourself. Nothing and nobody can sabotage your effort. You are stronger than your circumstances.

## MEAL 1: PRE-WORKOUT SNACK:
### Egg Whites + Pineapple Skin Infusion

See Egg Whites recipe on page 91 and Pineapple Skin Infusion recipe on page 212.

## MEAL 2: BREAKFAST:
### Turkey and Sun-Dried Tomato Omelette + Yucca Chips

**INGREDIENTS**

olive oil spray
1 tbsp chives, chopped
4 egg whites
2 slices turkey breast, low-fat
1 tsp sun-dried tomatoes, diced
salt to taste
pepper to taste
1 piece of cooked yucca (7½ oz)

**INSTRUCTIONS**

**1.** Place a nonstick skillet over medium heat and spray it with olive oil. Then sauté the chives for 1 minute.

**2.** Mix the eggs with the turkey breast and the dried tomatoes, and add to the skillet.

**3.** Mix slowly until cooked. Add salt and pepper and set aside.

**4.** For the yucca chips, use a mandoline to slice the piece of yucca finely. Place the slices on a perforated tray (such as those used to make pizza) and season with salt, pepper, and olive oil spray. Bake at 325°F for 25 minutes or until golden brown, making sure they don't burn.

**5.** Serve and enjoy.

**YIELD: 1 omelette (10.4 oz) + 0.9 oz yucca chips**

| 1,200-CALORIE PLAN | 1,500-CALORIE PLAN | 1,800-CALORIE PLAN |
|---|---|---|
| ▶ ½ omelette + 0.9 oz yucca chips | ▶ ¾ omelette + 0.9 oz yucca chips | ▶ 1 omelette + 0.9 oz yucca chips |

## MEAL 3: LUNCH:
**Grilled Chicken with Lemon and Sesame Cream + Vegetable Stir-Fry**

# grilled chicken with lemon and sesame cream

**INGREDIENTS**

2 skinless chicken breast fillets (16 oz)
pink Himalayan sea salt to taste
pepper to taste
½ tbsp tahini
1 tbsp lemon juice
½ tsp ground cumin
2 garlic cloves, crushed
½ cup water
olive oil spray
1 large white onion, julienned
1 cup leeks, julienned
½ cup parsley, chopped
1 tbsp lemon zest

**INSTRUCTIONS**

**1.** Season the chicken with salt and pepper.

**2.** Prepare the sesame cream by placing the tahini, lemon juice, cumin, garlic, and water in a food processor and processing until you obtain a homogenous cream. Set aside.

**3.** Add the chicken to a hot pan sprayed with olive oil and cook until it's browned on all sides. Set aside.

**4.** Preheat the oven to 375°F. Using the same frying pan in which you cooked the chicken, sauté the onion and the leeks until they are golden, without letting them burn.

*(Recipe continues)*

DAY 26

**5.** Place the chicken with onion and leeks in a baking dish.

**6.** Add the sesame cream and bake at 375°F for 15 minutes. Sprinkle with chopped parsley and lemon zest and serve.

YIELD: 20 oz

# vegetable stir-fry

### INGREDIENTS

olive oil spray
1 cup zucchini cut into half-moons
1 cup onion, julienned
1 cup red paprika, diced
1 cup yellow paprika, diced
1 cup mushrooms, chopped
1 cup green beans, chopped
pink Himalayan sea salt to taste
pepper to taste
fresh chives, finely chopped, to taste

### INSTRUCTIONS

**1.** Heat a wok over high heat and spray it with olive oil. While you wait for the pan to heat, season the vegetables with pink Himalayan sea salt and pepper.

**2.** Add the vegetables one at a time and sauté over high heat for about a minute each. Top with fresh chives and serve.

YIELD: 36.6 oz vegetables

| 1,200-CALORIE PLAN | 1,500-CALORIE PLAN | 1,800-CALORIE PLAN |
|---|---|---|
| ▶ 5 oz chicken with lemon sesame sauce + 1 cup vegetable stir-fry | ▶ 6 oz chicken with lemon sesame sauce + 1 cup vegetable stir-fry | ▶ 8.4 oz chicken with lemon sesame sauce + 1 cup vegetable stir-fry |

## MEAL 4: SNACK P.M. 1:
### Turkey, Arugula, and Tomato Eggplant Rolls

### INGREDIENTS

1 eggplant, sliced in half
salt to taste
pepper to taste
olive oil spray

2 slices turkey breast ham
½ cup arugula
1 tsp sun-dried tomatoes, diced

**INSTRUCTIONS**

**1.** Take an eggplant and, with the help of a sharp knife, cut it lengthwise to obtain 2 thin slices. Add salt and pepper.

**2.** Place a nonstick skillet over medium heat and spray it with olive oil. Grill the eggplant slices until browned.

**3.** Spread a slice on a plate and add a slice of turkey breast ham, half of the arugula, and half of the chopped sun-dried tomatoes and roll carefully. Repeat with the second slice.

**4.** Serve and enjoy.

YIELD: 2 rolls (1.9 oz each)

| 1,200-CALORIE PLAN | 1,500-CALORIE PLAN | 1,800-CALORIE PLAN |
|---|---|---|
| ▶1 roll | ▶1 roll | ▶2 rolls |

## MEAL 5: DINNER:
### Turkey Stew + Green Salad

# turkey stew
See recipe on page 131.

# green salad
See recipe on page 104.

| 1,200-CALORIE PLAN | 1,500-CALORIE PLAN | 1,800-CALORIE PLAN |
|---|---|---|
| ▶5.3 oz turkey chili + 1 cup green salad | ▶6.3 oz turkey chili + 1 cup green salad | ▶9 oz turkey chili + 1 cup green salad |

## MEAL 6: SNACK P.M. 2:
### Chocolate Chip Fit Protein Cupcake

See recipe on page 89.

**1,200-CALORIE PLAN**
▶ ½ cupcake

**1,500-CALORIE PLAN**
▶ 1 cupcake

**1,800-CALORIE PLAN**
▶ 1 cupcake*
*You can eat a maximum of 1½ cupcakes.

DAY 26

## Day 27

You're still shining. You're on your way. You've found your strength and you've proved to yourself that your motivation and your mind are much stronger than those dumbbells. Keep moving; every repetition makes you more beautiful, outside and in. It is a game of harmony, strength, and balance between what you eat, how much you rest, and how you train. The result is a strong, determined, and invincible woman.

## MEAL 1: PRE-WORKOUT SNACK:
### Egg Whites + Pineapple Skin Infusion

See Egg Whites recipe on page 91 and Pineapple Skin Infusion recipe on page 212.

## MEAL 2: BREAKFAST:
### Smoked Salmon and Avocado on Whole Wheat Toast

**INGREDIENTS**

2 slices of high-fiber whole wheat toast
4 slices of smoked salmon
¼ Hass avocado, finely sliced
1 tbsp sesame mayonnaise (1 tbsp Greek yogurt plus 1 tsp tahini plus lemon plus salt)
2 tsps fresh chives, chopped

**INSTRUCTIONS**

**1.** Take a piece of whole wheat toast and add a slice of smoked salmon, a slice of avocado, 1 teaspoon of sesame mayonnaise, and fresh chives.

**2.** Serve and enjoy.

YIELD: 2 slices of toast (4 oz each)

| 1,200-CALORIE PLAN | 1,500-CALORIE PLAN | 1,800-CALORIE PLAN |
|---|---|---|
| ▶ 1½ slices of toast | ▶ 2 slices of toast | ▶ 2½ slices of toast |

DAY 27

## MEAL 3: LUNCH:
**Turkey Stew + Mixed Salad with Avocado**

# turkey stew
See recipe on page 131.

# mixed salad with avocado
See recipe on page 224.

**1,200-CALORIE PLAN**
▶ 4.7 oz turkey chili + 1 bowl mixed salad with avocado

**1,500-CALORIE PLAN**
▶ 4.7 oz turkey chili + 1 bowl mixed salad with avocado

**1,800-CALORIE PLAN**
▶ 8 oz turkey chili + 1 bowl mixed salad with avocado

## MEAL 4: SNACK P.M. 1:
**Coconut Fit Protein Cupcake**

See recipe on page 89.

**1,200-CALORIE PLAN**
▶ ½ cupcake

**1,500-CALORIE PLAN**
▶ 1 cupcake

**1,800-CALORIE PLAN**
▶ 1 cupcake*
*You can eat a maximum of 1½ cupcakes.

## MEAL 5: DINNER:
**Sautéed Shrimp on Zucchini Noodles**

**INGREDIENTS**

3 large zucchini

1 tbsp olive oil

16 oz shrimp, cleaned and deveined

1 tbsp garlic, crushed

1 tsp powdered paprika

zest of 1 lemon

1 pinch of red pepper flakes

½ cup cherry tomatoes, cut into halves

pink Himalayan sea salt to taste

DAY 27

**pepper to taste**
**1 tbsp fresh parsley, finely chopped**

### INSTRUCTIONS

**1.** Zucchini noodles are made with the help of the special vegetable-noodle maker. If you don't have one, you can make the noodles by cutting long, thin slices with the help of a very sharp knife.

**2.** Place a large nonstick skillet over high heat and add the olive oil.

**3.** Season the shrimp with garlic, paprika, lemon zest, and red pepper flakes. Sauté until they brown on both sides.

**4.** Add the cherry tomatoes to the skillet and cook for a couple of minutes. Adjust the seasoning with the salt and pepper.

**5.** Add the raw zucchini noodles to the skillet, turn off the heat, and serve immediately with parsley.

YIELD: 24 oz

| 1,200-CALORIE PLAN | 1,500-CALORIE PLAN | 1,800-CALORIE PLAN |
|---|---|---|
| ▶ 4.8 oz | ▶ 5.7 oz | ▶ 8 oz |

## MEAL 6: SNACK P.M. 2:
### Chicken Stew + Eggplant Chips

## chicken stew

See recipe on page 131.

## eggplant chips

### INGREDIENTS

**10 eggplant slices**
**salt to taste**
**pepper to taste**
**olive oil spray**

### INSTRUCTIONS

**1.** Take an eggplant and, with the help of a sharp knife, cut it transversely into thin slices. Add salt and pepper to your liking.

*(Recipe continues)*

**DAY 27**

**2.** Place the eggplant slices on a baking sheet previously sprayed with olive oil, and bake at 325°F until golden brown. (You can also use an air fryer.)

**3.** Serve and enjoy.

**YIELD: 4 oz chicken stew + 10 eggplant chips**

| 1,200-CALORIE PLAN | 1,500-CALORIE PLAN | 1,800-CALORIE PLAN |
|---|---|---|
| ▶ 4 oz chicken stew + 10 eggplant chips | ▶ 5 oz chicken stew + 10 eggplant chips | ▶ 6 oz chicken stew + 10 eggplant chips |

DAY 27

## Day 28

Did you make it? How does it feel? Send me a message on my Instagram. Tell me everything. Do you feel powerful, happy, and self-confident? It's the explosion in your mind—the energy—that makes you feel invincible. Your new life has begun. Congratulations! You are a goddess. This is the first victory of many to come.

Rock and roll, baby! You did it!

## MEAL 1: PRE-WORKOUT SNACK:
**Egg Whites + Pineapple Skin Infusion**

See Egg Whites recipe on page 91 and Pineapple Skin Infusion recipe on page 212.

## MEAL 2: BREAKFAST:
**Eggs and Avocado on Brown Rice Crackers**

### INGREDIENTS

3 hard-boiled eggs, peeled (use only one yolk)
½ Hass avocado, small
1 tbsp sun-dried tomatoes, chopped
pink Himalayan sea salt to taste
chili pepper flakes to taste
2 brown rice crackers
1 tbsp chives

### INSTRUCTIONS

**1.** Crush the eggs with a fork and mix in the avocado, sun-dried tomatoes, salt, and chili pepper flakes to taste.

**2.** Serve over brown rice crackers and cover with some chives.

**YIELD: 14 oz eggs and avocado**

| 1,200-CALORIE PLAN | 1,500-CALORIE PLAN | 1,800-CALORIE PLAN |
|---|---|---|
| ► ½ serving of eggs with avocado + 1 rice cracker | ► ¾ serving of eggs with avocado + 2 rice crackers | ► 1 serving of eggs with avocado + 3 rice crackers |

# grilled chicken

### INGREDIENTS

16 oz whole chicken with skin and bone, piece of your choice

1 tbsp BBQ seasoning

1 tsp ginger, grated

1 tbsp Dijon mustard

1 tbsp Sweet-and-Sour Mustard (see recipe below)

1 stevia packet

1 clove garlic, crushed

zest and juice of 1 orange

1 tsp sriracha sauce

pink Himalayan sea salt to taste

### INSTRUCTIONS

**1.** Season the piece of chicken with the BBQ seasoning, ginger, Dijon mustard, sweet-and-sour mustard, stevia, garlic, orange zest, orange juice, and sriracha sauce, and place it in an airtight bag. Refrigerate for 6 hours.

**2.** Remove the chicken from the marinade, and add salt to taste.

**3.** Fire up the grill to high heat and grill the piece of chicken, browning it on all sides. Once it reaches the desired cooking point, remove it from the heat and let it stand.

# sweet-and-sour mustard

### INGREDIENTS

2 tbsps mustard

1 tbsp balsamic vinegar

1 tsp olive oil

1 stevia packet

pepper to taste

### INSTRUCTIONS

Mix all ingredients and serve.

DAY 28

# pineapple coleslaw salad

See recipe on page 168.

See recipe on page 168.

**1,200-CALORIE PLAN**
► 4 oz grilled chicken + 1 tbsp sweet-and-sour mustard + 1 cup pineapple coleslaw salad

**1,500-CALORIE PLAN**
► 5 oz grilled chicken + 1 tbsp sweet-and-sour mustard + 1 cup pineapple coleslaw salad

**1,800-CALORIE PLAN**
► 7 oz grilled chicken + 1 tbsp sweet-and-sour mustard + 1 cup pineapple coleslaw salad

## MEAL 4: SNACK P.M. 1:
### Green Apple or Pear + Peanut Butter

See recipe on page 193.

## MEAL 5: DINNER:
### Cheat Meal

## MEAL 6: SNACK P.M. 2:
### Chocolate Protein Ice Cream

**INGREDIENTS**

3 egg whites
1 tbsp cocoa powder
1 scoop of chocolate whey protein
1–2 stevia packets
2 tbsps Greek yogurt

**INSTRUCTIONS**

**1.** Using an electric mixer, beat the egg whites at high speed until they form soft peaks, about 2 minutes.

**2.** Bring the mixer to low speed and gradually add the cocoa, whey protein, stevia, and Greek yogurt.

**3.** Transfer the mixture to a separate container (such as a Popsicle mold) and allow it to cool in the freezer for 4 hours or until until it is firm.

**4.** Serve and enjoy.

YIELD: 1 cup (8 oz)

**1,200-CALORIE PLAN**
► ½ cup

**1,500-CALORIE PLAN**
► ½ cup

**1,800-CALORIE PLAN**
► 1 cup

DAY 28

# SUBSTITUTION PLAN

How can you repeat the plan, with its variations, until you reach your goal?

Now that you have completed the meal plan I designed specifically for you over the course of these twenty-eight days—and because you persisted and stayed motivated during these four weeks—it's time to CELEBRATE! You must be very proud of yourself, because I know it's not easy to make the decision to change your eating style and get rid of your bad habits—the bad habits that have made you overweight and tired and listless, the ones that have made you not feel satisfied with what you see in the mirror. Now that you have put into practice everything I've recommended, and now that you have followed this program to the very end, you have my absolute admiration and respect.

However, I know that we are not all the same, that the transformation process and the time it takes each and every one of us to reach our ideal weight varies depending on age, weight, lifestyle, physical activity, hormonal health, related diseases, and other factors. That's why I have created a "substitution plan," where I've included all the foods I eat in my daily diet. I have divided them into three groups according to their macronutrients (lean proteins, complex carbohydrates, and healthy fats), so that once you have completed your first twenty-eight-day plan and you want to repeat it to reach your goal, you can use these food options for as long as you like, until you reach your goal weight.

You need to choose the serving sizes associated with your calorie plan, and include one food from each group in each of your three main meals. Here are the DELICIOUS AND HEALTHY menu substitutions that you can use from now on—with variations and without having to eat the same things all the time—until you reach your goal!

## BREAKFAST ▶

| LEAN PROTEIN SOURCES | 1,200-CALORIE PLAN SUGGESTED SERVING | 1,500-CALORIE PLAN SUGGESTED SERVING | 1,800-CALORIE PLAN SUGGESTED SERVING |
|---|---|---|---|
| Eggs | 4.2 oz / 1 egg + 2 egg whites | 10.1 oz (1 egg + 4 egg whites) | 12.3 oz (2 eggs + 4 egg whites) |
| Chicken breast (shredded or ground) | 2.3 oz / ¾ cup | 3½ oz / 1 cup | 4.6 oz / 1¼ cups |
| Turkey breast (ground) | 2.3 oz / ¾ cup | 3½ oz / 1 cup | 4.6 oz / 1¼ cups |
| Natural tuna | 2.3 oz / ¾ cup | 3½ oz / 1 cup | 4.6 oz / 1¼ cups |
| Bison (ground) | 2.3 oz / ¾ cup | 3½ oz / 1 cup | 4.6 oz / 1¼ cups |
| Whey protein (your favorite flavor) | ½ oz / ½ scoop | 1 oz / 1 scoop | 1 oz / 1 scoop |
| Smoked salmon | 2.3 oz / 1 slice | 3½ oz / 1½ slices | 4.6 oz / 2 slices |
| Nonfat Greek yogurt, sugar-free | 5 oz / 1 cup + ½ serving of another lean protein source | 5 oz / 1 cup + ¾ serving of another lean protein source | 5 oz / 1 cup + ¾ serving of another lean protein source |
| COMPLEX CARBOHYDRATE SOURCES | 1,200-CALORIE PLAN SUGGESTED SERVING | 1,500-CALORIE PLAN SUGGESTED SERVING | 1,800-CALORIE PLAN SUGGESTED SERVING |
| Rolled oats | 3.4 oz / 1 cup | 5.1 oz / 1½ cups | 6.8 oz / 2 cups |
| Oat bran | 1.6 oz / ½ cup | 2½ oz / ¾ cup | 3.3 oz / 1 cup |
| Yellow plantain, parboiled | 3.3 oz / 1 small unit | 5 oz / 1½ small units | 6.6 oz / 2 small units |
| Green plantain, parboiled | 3.3 oz / 1 small unit | 5 oz / 1 medium unit | 6.6 oz / 1 large unit |
| Sweet potatoes, yams, cooked | 4.3 oz / 1 small unit | 6½ oz / 1 medium unit | 8.6 oz / 1 large unit |
| Wheat-germ bread | 1 oz / 2 slices | 1½ oz / 3 slices | 2 oz / 4 slices |
| Pumpkin | 2½ oz / ½ cup + ¾ serving of another complex carbohydrate source | 5 oz / 1 cup + ¾ serving of another complex carbohydrate source | 5 oz / 1 cup + ¾ serving of another complex carbohydrate source |
| Carrots | 2 oz / ½ small unit + ¾ serving of another complex carbohydrate source | 4 oz / 1 small unit + ¾ serving of another complex carbohydrate source | 4 oz / 1 small unit + ¾ serving of another complex carbohydrate source |
| Potato, raw or cooked | 6.6 oz / 1 medium unit | 8.3 oz / 1½ medium units | 13.3 oz / 2 medium units |
| Quinoa arepa | 6 oz / 1 medium unit | 7.3 oz / 1 large unit | 8.6 oz / 2 small units |
| Oatmeal arepa | 6 oz / 1 medium unit | 7.3 oz / 1 large unit | 8.6 oz / 2 small units |

*(Table continues)*

| COMPLEX CARBOHYDRATE SOURCES | 1,200-CALORIE PLAN SUGGESTED SERVING | 1,500-CALORIE PLAN SUGGESTED SERVING | 1,800-CALORIE PLAN SUGGESTED SERVING |
|---|---|---|---|
| Yucca arepa | 4.3 oz / 1 small unit | 5.6 oz / 1 medium unit | 7 oz / 1 large unit |
| Multigrain arepa | 6 oz / 1 medium unit | 7.3 oz / 1 large unit | 8.6 oz / 2 small units |
| Brown rice or pocorn crackers | ½ oz / 3 units | 1 oz / up to 6 units | 1½ oz / up to 6 units |
| High-fiber whole wheat toast | 0.9 oz / 2 slices | 1.4 oz / 3 slices | 1.8 oz / 4 slices |
| Oatmeal pancakes | 3 oz / 1½ pancakes | 4 oz / 2 pancakes | 6 oz / 3 pancakes |

| HEALTHY FAT SOURCES | 1,200-CALORIE PLAN SUGGESTED SERVING | 1,500-CALORIE PLAN SUGGESTED SERVING | 1,800-CALORIE PLAN SUGGESTED SERVING |
|---|---|---|---|
| Avocado | 2.3 oz / 2 medium slices | 3½ oz / 3 medium slices | 4.6 oz / 4 medium slices |
| Unsalted peanuts | ½ oz / 20 units | ¾ oz / 30 units | 1 oz / 40 units |
| Almonds or cashews | 0.8 oz / 12 units | 1.2 oz / 18 units | 1.6 oz / 24 units |
| Natural nut butters | 0.8 oz / 1 tbsp | 0.8 oz / 1 tbsp | 1.2 oz / 1½ tbsps |
| Almond flour | 0.8 oz / ¼ cup | 1 oz / ⅓ cup | 1 oz / ⅓ cup |
| Extra-virgin olive oil or coconut oil | 0.3 oz / ½ tbsp | ½ oz / 1 tbsp | 0.7 oz / 1½ tbsps |
| Black olives | 1 oz / up to 4 units | 1½ oz / up to 6 units | 2 oz / up to 8 units |

## LUNCH ▶

| LEAN PROTEIN SOURCES | 1,200-CALORIE PLAN SUGGESTED SERVING | 1,500-CALORIE PLAN SUGGESTED SERVING | 1,800-CALORIE PLAN SUGGESTED SERVING |
|---|---|---|---|
| Bluefish: fresh salmon, tuna, sardine, sea trout, mullet, eel, swordfish, lamprey, turbot | 4 oz / 1 medium fillet | 5 oz / 1 large fillet | 7 oz / 2 medium fillets |
| Whitefish: tilapia, dorado, grouper, mackerel, hake, corvina, lisa, sea bass, bonito, snapper, others | 5.8 oz / 2 small fillets | 7 oz / 3 small fillets | 10 oz / 2 large fillets |
| Seafood: prawns, shrimp, mussels, scallops, clams, lobster, squid, octopus | 4 oz / 1 cup | 5 oz / 1¼ cup | 7 oz / 1¾ cups |
| Chicken breast | 4 oz / 1 small breast | 5 oz / 1 medium breast | 7 oz / 1 large breast |
| Turkey breast (ground) | 4 oz / 1 cup | 5 oz / 1¼ cups | 7 oz / 1¾ cups |
| Beef tenderloin | 4 oz / 1 small steak | 5 oz / 1 medium steak | 7 oz / 2 small steaks |
| Bison (ground) | 4 oz / 1 cup | 5 oz / 1¼ cups | 7 oz / 1¾ cups |
| Pork loin | 4 oz / 2 slices | 5 oz / 2½ slices | 7 oz / 3½ slices |

| COMPLEX CARBOHYDRATE SOURCES | 1,200-CALORIE PLAN SUGGESTED SERVING | 1,500-CALORIE PLAN SUGGESTED SERVING | 1,800-CALORIE PLAN SUGGESTED SERVING |
|---|---|---|---|
| Brown rice | 2.1 oz / ½ cup | 4.2 oz | 6.3 oz |
| Quinoa | 2.1 oz / ½ cup | 4.2 oz | 6.3 oz |
| Yellow plantain, parboiled | 1.6 oz / ½ small unit | 3.3 oz | 5 oz |
| Green plantain, parboiled | 3.3 oz / 1 small unit | 3.3 oz | 5 oz |
| Sweet potato, cooked | 2.1 oz / ½ unit | 4.2 oz | 6.3 oz |
| Potato, cooked | 3.3 oz / ½ unit | 6.6 oz | 9.9 oz |
| Yucca, cooked | 1.3 oz / ⅓ cup | 2.6 oz / ⅔ cup | 3.9 oz / 1 cup |
| Legumes: lentils, peas, beans, chickpeas, others | 3.3 oz / ½ cup | 6.6 oz | 9.9 oz |
| High-fiber whole wheat toast | ½ oz / 1 slice | 1 oz | 1½ oz |

*(Table continues)*

| HEALTHY FAT SOURCES | 1,200-CALORIE PLAN SUGGESTED SERVING | 1,500-CALORIE PLAN SUGGESTED SERVING | 1,800-CALORIE PLAN SUGGESTED SERVING |
| --- | --- | --- | --- |
| Avocado | 2.3 oz / 2 medium slices | 3½ oz / 3 medium slices | 4.6 oz / 4 medium slices |
| Extra-virgin olive oil, coconut oil | 0.3 oz / ½ tbsp | ½ oz / 1 tbsp | 0.7 oz / 1½ tbsps |
| Black olives | 1 oz / up to 4 units | 1½ oz / up to 6 units | 2 oz / up to 8 units |

## DINNER ▶

| LEAN PROTEIN SOURCES | 1,200-CALORIE PLAN SUGGESTED SERVING | 1,500-CALORIE PLAN SUGGESTED SERVING | 1,800-CALORIE PLAN SUGGESTED SERVING |
|---|---|---|---|
| Bluefish: fresh salmon, tuna, sardine, sea trout, mullet, eel, swordfish, lamprey, turbot | 4 oz / 1 medium fillet | 5 oz / 1 large fillet | 7 oz / 2 medium fillets |
| Whitefish: tilapia, dorado, grouper, mackerel, hake, corvina, lisa, sea bass, bonito, snapper, others | 5.8 oz / 2 small fillets | 7 oz / 3 small fillets | 10 oz / 2 large fillets |
| Seafood: prawns, shrimp, mussels, scallops, clams, lobster, squid, octopus | 4 oz / 1 cup | 5 oz / 1¼ cups | 7 oz / 1¾ cups |
| Chicken breast | 4 oz / 1 small breast | 5 oz / 1 medium breast | 7 oz / 1 large breast |
| Turkey breast (ground) | 4 oz / 1 cup | 5 oz / 1¼ cups | 7 oz / 1¾ cups |
| Beef tenderloin | 4 oz / 1 small steak | 5 oz / 1 medium steak | 7 oz / 2 small steaks |
| Bison (ground) | 4 oz / 1 cup | 5 oz / 1¼ cups | 7 oz / 1¾ cups |
| Pork loin | 4 oz / 2 slices | 5 oz / 2½ slices | 7 oz / 3½ slices |
| HEALTHY FAT SOURCES | 1,200-CALORIE PLAN SUGGESTED SERVING | 1,500-CALORIE PLAN SUGGESTED SERVING | 1,800-CALORIE PLAN SUGGESTED SERVING |
| Avocado | 2.3 oz / 2 medium slices | 3½ oz / 3 medium slices | 4.6 oz / 4 medium slices |
| Extra-virgin olive oil or coconut oil | 0.3 oz / ½ tbsp | ½ oz / 1 tbsp | 0.7 oz / 1½ tbsps |
| Black olives | 1 oz / up to 4 units | 1½ oz / up to 6 units | 2 oz / up to 8 units |

I suggest including vegetables in all your main meals, and at lunch and dinner have them occupy half your plate, whether they're steamed, baked, grilled, or in a salad. Include at least five different vegetables; season them with lemon, extra-virgin olive oil, vinegar, pepper, and your favorite spices.

## PERMITTED VEGETABLES

- Artichokes
- Leeks
- Eggplants
- Watercress
- Broccoli
- Zucchini
- Onions, green onions, or scallions
- White onions
- Purple or red onions
- Chives
- Celery
- Mushrooms
- Chayote
- Cilantro
- Brussels sprouts
- Cauliflower
- Asparagus
- Spinach
- Escarole
- Endive
- Fennel
- Kale
- Romaine lettuce
- Chinese turnip
- Hearts of palm
- Cucumbers
- Parsley
- Bell peppers
- Portobello mushrooms
- Japanese radish or daikon
- Cabbage
- Purple cabbage
- Radicchio
- Arugula
- Tomatoes or Roma tomatoes
- Cherry tomatoes

| FRUIT SOURCES (SIMPLE CARBOHYDRATES) | 1,200-CALORIE PLAN SUGGESTED SERVING | 1,500-CALORIE PLAN SUGGESTED SERVING | 1,800-CALORIE PLAN SUGGESTED SERVING |
|---|---|---|---|
| Blueberries, cherries, blackberries, strawberries, or red berries | 2.6 oz / 4 units | 5.3 oz / 8 units | 7.8 oz / 12 units |
| Plums | 16 oz / ½ unit | 3.3 oz / 1 unit | 4.8 oz / 1½ units |
| Peaches | 2.1 oz / 1 unit | 4.3 oz / 1½ units | 6.3 oz / 2 units |
| Guavas | 5½ oz / ½ unit | 11 oz / 1½ units | 15.6 oz / 2 units |
| Kiwis | 2 oz / ½ unit | 4 oz / 1 medium unit | 6 oz / 1½ medium units |
| Mandarins | 3.4 oz / ½ large unit | 6.7 oz / 1 large unit | 10.2 oz / 1½ large units |
| Green and red apples | 2.7 oz / 1 small unit | 5.3 oz / 1 medium unit | 8.1 oz / 1 large unit |
| Mangoes | 2 oz / ½ medium unit | 4 oz / 1 medium unit | 6 oz / 1 large unit |

| FRUIT SOURCES (SIMPLE CARBOHYDRATES) | 1,200-CALORIE PLAN SUGGESTED SERVING | 1,500-CALORIE PLAN SUGGESTED SERVING | 1,800-CALORIE PLAN SUGGESTED SERVING |
|---|---|---|---|
| Melons | 8 oz / ¾ cup | 16 oz / 1¼ cups | 24 oz / 2½ cups |
| Nectarines | 1½ oz / ½ large unit | 3 oz / 1 large unit | 4½ oz / 1½ large units |
| Oranges | 4.1 oz / ½ medium unit | 8.3 oz / 1 medium unit | 12.3 oz / 1½ medium units |
| Pears | 4 oz / ½ unit | 8 oz / 1 unit | 12 oz / 1½ units |
| Pineapples | 1.6 oz / 1 small slice | 3.3 oz / 1½ small slices | 4.8 oz / 2 small slices |
| Raisins | 0.3 oz / 10 units | 0.6 oz / 20 units | 0.9 oz / 30 units |
| Grapefruit | 12.3 oz / ½ unit | 18.4 oz / ¾ unit | 24.6 oz / 1 unit |

## THE FRUITS I RECOMMEND

If you are going to include fruit at breakfast, here's how I suggest you incorporate it:

1. **As a main carbohydrate:** Eat twice the portion suggested in the above table, of the fruit of your choice, according to the calorie plan you are following. If you are going to combine two fruits, then take the suggested portion of each.

2. **As part of a carbohydrate:** Eat the portion suggested in this table of the fruit of your choice, according to the calorie plan you are following. Add three-quarters of the suggested portion of the carbohydrate of your choice in the "breakfast" table.

3. If possible, eat all fruits with their skin in order to increase the fiber content. Don't consume fruits in the form of simple juices.

# 8.

# MAINTENANCE: IT'S NOT A PLAN; IT'S A LIFESTYLE

**T**here is nothing worse than feeling limited. The very word *diet* sounds like a jail, obligation, and restriction. But it's a word that has long been misused. The word actually means "life regimen," and it has to do with what you tend to eat on a regular basis. Now that you have learned what it takes to change your body and your life, I'm going to ask you to forget the word *diet* and replace it with "my healthy habits." Tell your mind and body that no one is forcing you to do anything, that these habits are good for you and you have chosen them freely. And that will make a big difference. Repeat the mantra that these habits are good for you and that you have chosen them. Do it for a while and you will see that you will never have to "diet" again in order to fix the excesses of the past. Now that you have the knowledge, all you have to do is put it into practice, day after day. Fill your life with positive habits. It's easy—you just have to do the right thing every day, one day at a time.

. . .

# THE GOLDEN RULES TO CHANGING YOUR HABITS

## 1. GET OFF THAT ROLLER COASTER—NOW!

If you fall into temptation, stop right away. We are all human and some-times we fall into temptation—it has happened to me too! But what has made the difference in this journey I have undertaken is that I have the ability to stop and not continue eating poorly for the rest of the day or the week. This is one of the things that has allowed me to continue to enjoy this lifestyle and its rewards on a daily basis.

And how do I do it? Simple: I stay focused on my goals. And I know that for every day I let myself down, I will be one day further away from reaching them. So, I want you to take this advice and apply it from now on: you are going to allow yourself to keep what you have achieved here for the rest of your life. You aren't going to be just another one of the millions of girls who are frustrated because they want to change their bodies and improve their weight but don't ever achieve lasting results. So get off that roller coaster—now!

## 2. HE WHO SINS AND PRAYS EVENS THE SCORE

There is a Colombian proverb, *"El que peca y reza empata,"* which rough-ly translates as "He who sins and prays evens the score." Which leads me to the question: Did you eat something you shouldn't be eating? Take action that day or the next day, period. Whenever you eat something outside your usual diet or fall into temptation, compensate for it the next day by doing more cardio, eating fewer carbs, and training harder. Soon enough you'll "even the score."

## 3. IF YOU CAN'T EAT IT, DON'T BUY IT!

Do not buy or have anything around the house that can sabotage your diet. This simple trick will allow you to eat only foods that are good for you, even in times of anxiety or stress. One of my secrets to controlling my cravings is to eat popcorn and berries, because they satisfy me and it makes me feel good to know that I can eat something delicious while still watching my figure and my diet.

## 4. SIZE DOES MATTER!

I've said it a thousand times, but I don't want you to forget it so I'll say it again: you have to control your portion size while you're on this plan but you also need to continue to do it for the rest of your life. Just as important as the quality of what you eat is how much you eat. For example, I adjust my portions to four ounces of protein every three hours and I accompany them with carbs or vegetables depending on the case.

## 5. ALWAYS VARY YOUR ROUTINE!

If you exercise on the elliptical machine every day or do the same workout, there comes a time when your body ceases to react. It becomes accustomed to what you are doing and you get stuck. That's why you have to change up your training routine (I do it every week). The same goes for your metabolism: if you give it the same type of food from Monday to Monday, without changing anything, there will come a time when you will enter an adaptive state, and your metabolism will slow down. That's why I recommend that you switch your diet up every day (as shown in my menu plan) and that you give yourself a cheat meal once a week if you want to keep seeing your body change.

## 6. MAKE IT A PART OF YOUR LIFE!

I'm already disciplined, and this lifestyle is inside me. It's my routine; it's like brushing my teeth. I go to the gym twice a day whether or not I have the time, because it's part of my job. Making this a part of my life was not easy, I wasn't always very focused, and there were ups and downs . . . but once I decided that this was what I was going to do and I started to see and enjoy the results, I started to live and feel like it was a part of my life. You too can do it; you just have to start, be consistent, and wait for the changes, and little by little your body will begin to recognize it as a part of your life too.

# HOW DO YOU MAINTAIN YOUR GOAL WEIGHT?

Did you reach your goal weight? Don't let it go! If you have already arrived here and managed to get to the body you so desperately wanted, let me tell you that the next step in your journey is so much easier. What matters is that you keep watching what you eat and never go back.

Once you have reached your goal, my recommendation is:

1. Return and take the test in chapter seven to determine the number of calories you should consume based on your basal metabolic rate, age, and level of physical activity. Once you have the result leave it as it is, without subtracting or adding anything, because this time your goal will be to maintain your current weight.

2. Depending on the number you have obtained as a result, select the calorie plan that you must follow from now on (it should be the one closest to that result). Also, remember that you have a substitution plan that will allow you to vary your menus without ever getting bored.

3. You can have a cheat meal once a week: if you have already achieved the body you want and don't want to lose any more weight, I recommend that you take a meal off once a week, so that you can stay focused and 100 percent on track and following your diet plan and exercise routine during the rest of the week.

4. Stay active, and exercise five to six times a week.

5. Apply the golden rules I just shared with you, because they will allow you to change your habits forever.

# WHAT TO DO WHEN EATING OUT?

First of all, choose the restaurant where you are going to eat. Restaurants that specialize in meats, fish, or seafood—such as steak houses, seafood restaurants, or Japanese restaurants—are excellent options. I suggest eating a serving of lean protein, roasted or baked, with a large bowl of vegetables or raw salad with the dressing on the side or a simple dressing of olive oil, vinegar, lemon, and pepper. Accompany with water or some natural infusion without sugar.

Here are some slightly more specific recommendations depending on the type of restaurant you visit:

- At a **Japanese restaurant**, order edamame or a simple seaweed salad (wakame). Avoid adding soy sauce to your meals. Order sashimi, tartares, and fresh fish rolls without rice or cream cheese, and accompany with lemon green tea, without sugar. I also love ordering an Asian fish or seafood soup before the main course.

- At a **Chinese restaurant**, select a main dish that includes a grilled or steamed protein (and that isn't fried or covered in a thick sweet-and-sour sauce) with abundant vegetables (avoid selecting sautéed vegetables, because of their high oil and soy content). Accompany with water or some natural infusion without sugar.

- At a **Peruvian restaurant**, select fish or seafood ceviches, as well as fish *tiraditos* in all their shapes and colors. Although we know these dishes have a slightly high sodium content (salt), the fact is that it's only sodium and you'll be able to expel it easily the next day. Other options that you can select are sautéed tenderloin, *aguadito de gallina*, seafood *escabeche*, and *choros a la chalaca*. Accompany with water or some natural infusion without sugar.

- At an **Italian restaurant**, you can order a carpaccio or a fresh salad (forget the Caesar salad). If you're in the mood for pasta, make sure it is whole wheat and al dente, with a red sauce containing proteins and vegetables (avoid white cream- or cheese-based sauces). Eat only one-fourth of the pasta dish, and accompany with a serving of protein (salmon, whitefish, or chicken) and a bowl of fresh salad with vinaigrette and olive oil. Avoid eating the bread with olive oil that is brought to the table while you wait. Accompany with water or some natural infusion without sugar.

- At a **Mexican restaurant**, stay away from the *totopos* (fried corn chips) and the sauces they give you while you wait. Order a broth-based soup, a ceviche, or even a simple nopal salad. Select a main course containing protein and pico de gallo garnish, a raw salad, and guacamole (don't go overboard with the guacamole, though, since it is a high-fat preparation). You can order fajitas, for example, and eat them without the tortilla. Accompany with water or some natural infusion without sugar.

▶ At a **Middle Eastern or Greek restaurant**, select chicken or beef kebabs as your main protein accompanied by a tabbouleh or *fattoush* salad, or vegetables such as eggplants, onions, zucchini, and peppers. You can accompany them with cucumber yogurt dip (tzatziki), hummus (chickpea dip), eggplant, and red pepper dip, but always in moderation (no more than two tablespoons). Avoid eating the Middle Eastern bread or the fried chips they offer while you wait at the table. If you get the kibbe or falafel, ask for it to be baked. If you want a shawarma, skip the bread. Accompany with water or some natural infusion without sugar.

▶ If you go to any other kind of restaurant serving international food, do the following:

- Don't go hungry. Eat a light snack before you leave.
- Avoid ordering an appetizer, and stay away from the bread basket.
- Select dishes with few ingredients, unless they are vegetables.
- Ask the waiter to bring you the dish you selected without the sides (in the case of rice, mashed potatoes, risotto, pasta, steamed potatoes, and so on). Instead, order an extra serving of salad or steamed vegetables.
- If you notice that the portions of the dish you ordered exceed the ones you should normally consume, then share it with someone else or ask to take the rest home with you and give it away!
- Eat slowly and talk!
- Always drink water or natural infusions without sugar.
- Never order dessert. If you're craving something sweet, you can order coffee or some fruit.

# WHAT CAN YOU DO IF YOU GO ON A TRIP WHILE ON THIS PLAN?

Travel is a time of great risk, unless you act with intelligence and foresight. When I'm traveling I never lose my focus or neglect my food or my exercise routines. On the contrary, I do everything much better.

If you don't want a trip to ruin your weight-loss plan, never forget the following "fit" tips:

1. Don't skip meals. Organize your itineraries so you can eat your meals at the right times. Make sure you do at least three main meals and two snacks.
2. Never head out without a bottle of water and some healthy snack in your backpack. Fruits are excellent choices!
3. Plan your meals and restaurant visits. Don't improvise, because when you're hungry it's impossible to think.
4. Restrict complex carbohydrates; eat only fruits and lots of vegetables.
5. Eat lean or low-fat proteins (eggs, meats, fish, poultry, whey protein) in your three main meals and snacks.
6. Eat very clean and natural foods; don't eat anything processed.
7. Avoid eating grains, cereals, legumes, sugar and sugary foods, and products containing gluten and dairy, as well as fast food.
8. Exercise every day. In addition to maintaining my exercise routine, I get to know the cities I travel to by riding a bicycle or walking around.

Brick by brick you can build a very large wall. The same is true when it comes to your body. Every healthy habit, every exercise session, every bite you eat either brings you closer or draws you away from that fabulous version of yourself that you have visualized. Your habits shape your present and future life. If you want to have something good tomorrow, you have to start building today.

In the next chapter you will see that we have a bunch of allies that will help us to fulfill our goals. They will be a new healthy habit that you must incorporate into your morning routine. And so we change your life, your figure, and your destiny. Stay with me. We are going to take this to the next level.

# 9.

# SUPPLEMENTS: SUPER FRIENDS TO THE RESCUE!

**N**owadays people believe they can solve everything without having to put in any effort. Sometimes I laugh when I read on social media or in magazines certain comments that promise an instant change if you take a certain pill or dietary supplement. It saddens me to know that some girls fall into the deception of such products and end up more frustrated than when they started training, which only results in a waste of time, effort, and money. The truth is that instant gratification simply doesn't exist in the fitness world. If you want to change, you're going to have to put in the work and keep at it. There's no other way. That's why I want to talk about supplements—what they are, how I use them, and what they can truly do for you.

We know that nutrition and training are the big players when it comes to burning fat, gaining muscle, or improving performance. But from medical studies we have also learned that an intelligent and well-planned supplementation regimen can lead us to achieve the results we are looking for, faster. That's why in this chapter I want to share with you which nutritional supplements can help you improve your body composition and your physical performance.

But beware! You need to keep in mind that your specific needs will depend on the type of activity you do, the intensity and frequency with which you do it, and your particular goals.

**What are you looking for? Weight loss, increased muscle mass, or to increase your physical performance?**

There are useful supplements for each of these particular cases. To clear up any confusion, we will share a serious and systematic review of the supplements that are most used to lose weight, gain muscle mass, and increase performance, and we will look at the risks and benefits of these products. I don't intend to recommend exactly what supplements you should take—only your doctor or nutritionist should do that—but I am sharing the supplements that I have studied with my coauthor and doctor, Samar Yorde, and that have worked for me. I share information about only the supplements that seem to be effective, meaning that research studies have shown their efficacy and safety.

## SUPPLEMENTS I SHARE IN THIS CHAPTER:

**To Increase Muscle Mass**
- ▶ Proteins: muscle builders
- ▶ Amino Acids and BCAA: protein bricks
- ▶ Creatine: more strength, more muscle

**To Lose Weight**
- ▶ Thermogenics: the power of caffeine
- ▶ Green Tea: does it help you spend more energy?
- ▶ Conjugated Linoleic Acid (CLA)
- ▶ Calcium

**To Improve Performance**
- ▶ Carbohydrates and Electrolytes
- ▶ L-carnitine: the controversy

**Other Amino Acids: L-arginine and L-glutamine**

**Vitamins and Minerals: Invisible Heroes**

**Omega-3 Fatty Acids: Heart Health**

# SUPPLEMENTS FOR INCREASING MUSCLE MASS

## PROTEINS: MUSCLE BUILDERS

The amount of protein you need in order to increase and maintain your muscle mass when you follow an intense training routine is greater than the one recommended for a sedentary person, which is about one gram per kilogram of body weight per day (that means 60 grams if you weigh 60 kilograms). Most athletes and people who practice strength training may need up to 2 grams per kilogram per day (120 grams for a 60-kilogram person).

Although you should always try to cover these amounts with food, when your protein requirement is very high, it may be convenient to use a supplement to cover those extra needs. It has been proven that the optimal amount of protein to stimulate muscle recovery after a strength-training session is between twenty and twenty-five grams, the same amount usually contained in a scoop of any protein supplement.

However, the ideal time to consume it will depend on your particular training routine. For example, consuming a whey protein supplement with a serving of fruit thirty to sixty minutes before training might be a good idea if it's been many hours since your last meal, or if it's the first thing in the morning and you don't have the time to eat a full breakfast. However, if you finish training and your next meal isn't going to be for a couple of hours, you can consume a protein supplement immediately after your workout. When using casein (a slow-absorption protein), it is best to consume it between meals or before you go to bed.

Once we understand this, we realize that using protein supplements is not just about consuming protein after training, but knowing how to properly plan the *total* amount of protein in your daily diet, because even if you're taking the best supplement in the world, if the rest of your diet doesn't cover your daily protein needs, you're wasting your time (and your money). Ideally, you should have the guidance of a professional who's an expert on the topic and can help you plan the times at which you consume your protein according to your individual training routine in order to get the most out of it.

## AMINO ACIDS AND BCAAS: PROTEIN BRICKS

Surely you have heard or read all about them. The famous branched-chain amino acids (leucine, isoleucine, and valine), also known as BCAAs, are protein components that help stop muscle destruction and stimulate repair. Of these three amino acids, leucine, in particular, directly promotes muscle formation and plays an important role in the control of protein metabolism.

You can supplement daily with 8 to 12 grams of leucine or 12 to 18 grams of BCAA, divided into two doses of 4 to 5 grams before and/or after training. In fact, if your training session is very long, you can even take them during your session, since your muscles will use them as a direct source of energy. In any case, before considering taking an amino acid supplement, you must be clear that amino acids are already present in the proteins we consume, just likes bricks in a wall, so it could be redundant if you take a protein supplement and an amino acid at the same time.

In fact, whey protein supplements generally contain about four to five grams of BCAA per scoop.

## CREATINE: MORE STRENGTH, MORE MUSCLE

Creatine monohydrate is the safest and most effective supplement if you are looking to increase your strength and gain a few pounds of muscle. Simply put, it is the main fuel for strength and power workouts in which each movement lasts for a few seconds (for example, in weight lifting or sprinting).

We can obtain it naturally in foods such as meat, but in very small quantities, so supplementation is of great help. The fastest protocol for increasing creatine muscle stores is to consume 0.3 gram daily for each kilogram of weight for at least three days (about 20 grams daily if you weigh 70 kilograms) in what is known as the loading phase. From then on you can consume approximately 5 grams per day (the equivalent of a teaspoon), in what we call the maintenance phase. Many experts consider that the loading phase is not strictly necessary and one can go right ahead and start with 5 grams per day.

On the other hand, ideally, creatine should be consumed along with carbs and/or proteins for faster absorption. Although it was long recommended for before training, a recent study showed that it does a better job at increasing muscle mass and strength when consumed immediately after training. Either way, creatine is an excellent supplement if you are looking to gain muscle naturally and safely.

## SUPPLEMENTS FOR WEIGHT LOSS

### THERMOGENICS: THE POWER OF CAFFEINE

Thermogenics, known colloquially as pre-workouts or fat burners, are supplements that stimulate our central nervous system thanks to substances such as caffeine or green tea, allowing us to train more intensely and thus burn more calories. The main ingredient of thermogenics, caffeine, is one of the few supplements to have been shown to have a positive effect on physical performance, helping decrease perceived exertion.

It has been demonstrated that when consumed in moderate doses of 3 to 6 milligrams per kilogram of weight (for example, 180 to 360 milligrams if you weigh 60 kilograms), between 30 and 60 minutes before exercise, a caffeine supplement can improve performance in both short- and long-lasting activities. Thermogenics usually contain moderate doses of caffeine (100 to 400 milligrams). Doses greater than 3 to 6 milligrams per kilogram are unnecessary and have no additional benefits.

Now for the question you are probably asking yourself: is that coffee I drink in the morning or before training just as effective? The answer is somewhat disappointing: no. Although we can find caffeine in coffee, tea, and energy drinks, the doses are too low. For example, one cup of black coffee contains about 100 milligrams of caffeine (a dose that would be lower than 2 grams per kilogram in a 60-to-70-kilogram person). Also, if you are already a regular consumer of coffee, you will probably see fewer benefits. It is important that before using any thermogenic supplement, you consult with your doctor to make sure it's safe for you.

### GREEN TEA: DOES IT HELP YOU TO SPEND MORE ENERGY?

Nowadays green tea, similarly to caffeine, is one of the most common supplements found in weight-loss products, because it has been suggested that it helps burn fat. Green tea contains large amounts of substances called catechins, of which epigallocatechin gallate (EGCG), when combined with a low-calorie diet, has been associated with a possible increase in energy expenditure during the day. So, theoretically, this increase in energy expenditure could help you lose fat or improve your body composition, but unfortunately, so far there is not enough evidence to support this theory.

### CONJUGATED LINOLEIC ACID (CLA)

CLA is also an essential fatty acid of the omega-3 series, with a slightly modified structure. It seems to decrease body fat accumulation significantly, due to its apparent ability to improve the effect of insulin at muscle level.

The daily consumption recommendation is one thousand milligrams of CLA twice a day, with breakfast and dinner. So far, there are no known side effects or contraindications.

### CALCIUM

Some research has suggested that supplementation with calcium (800 milligrams per day) or high intake of this mineral through diet (1,200 to 1,300 milligrams per day) may stimulate fat loss compared to a low-calcium diet (400 to 500 milligrams per day). However, further study is needed in relation to calcium supplementation to be able to issue definitive conclusions.

## SUPPLEMENTS FOR IMPROVING PHSYICAL PERFORMANCE

### CARBOHYDRATES AND ELECTROLYTES

One of the most critical points of training is being able to stay hydrated and recover not only water but also the carbohydrates and electrolytes lost to sweating, especially in hot or humid environments. If your workouts are of low to moderate intensity and they last for less than an hour, you can perfectly hydrate yourself with water. But after ninety minutes, or if your workout is very intense, carbohydrate deficiency and sodium losses become significant (those white spots on your clothes after a long workout are actually the salts you lose when you sweat). Only in these cases is it a good idea to consume during training, in addition to water, a source of carbohydrates and electrolytes such as sports drinks (500 to 1,000 cubic centimeters per hour) or carbohydrate gels (1 to 2 gels per hour) to prevent dehydration and maintain your performance.

## L-CARNITINE: THE CONTROVERSY

L-carnitine is undoubtedly one of the most common components found in weight-loss supplements. It is an important cellular transporter of fats. Put simply, each molecule of L-carnitine inside our cells would be a kind of truck that takes the garbage (fat) from the landfill (cytoplasm) to the furnaces (mitochondria) to be burned (oxidized).

Unfortunately, the vast majority of research so far has shown that supplementation with L-carnitine has no effect on the amount of carnitine in the muscles (that is, the "trucks" that you bring in from the outside will have no work to do), or on fat metabolism, weight loss, or sports performance. But not all the news is discouraging—other recent studies have shown that L-carnitine supplementation may have a minimal effect on the reduction of exercise-induced oxidative stress, which may help athletes to tolerate training with greater intensity.

# OTHER AMINO ACIDS: L-ARGININE AND L-GLUTAMINE

Both L-arginine and L-glutamine are amino acids that, although ineffective when we are looking to increase muscle mass, lose fat, or improve physical performance, provide some health benefits that could justify supplementation in some cases.

L-glutamine helps us to form new proteins, to heal better, to maintain the acid-base balance, and to strengthen our immune system. In addition, it is a source of energy. You can supplement in doses of 8 to 12 grams a day in separate doses. L-arginine is involved in cell division, healing, immune system functioning, and ammonia elimination, and it helps control blood pressure. It can be supplemented in doses of 10 to 14 grams per day in separate doses.

## VITAMINS AND MINERALS: INVISIBLE HEROES

A large percentage of the population of the United States has deficiencies in many vitamins and minerals due to poor lifestyle habits and consuming food that has inadequate amounts of these nutrients.

Athletes, in particular, are a population prone to nutritional deficiencies because we have much higher requirements than sedentary people. This is why it is currently recommended that athletes consume multivitamins that contain between 300 and 600 percent of the recommended daily values (DV) for most vitamins and minerals, in order to meet the high nutritional requirements of intense training, especially when we are on a low-calorie diet in order to lose body fat.

Another important point is that you should not consider supplementing with specific vitamins or minerals (for example, vitamin C, folic acid, calcium, or iron) without first consulting with your nutritionist or your doctor.

## OMEGA-3 FATTY ACIDS: HEART HEALTH

Omega-3 fatty acids are necessary for the normal functioning of your cells and organs, and they are present in each of the cells of your body. It is estimated that more than eighty thousand people die prematurely each year in the United States as a result of a deficiency of these essential fats. Vegetarians, in particular, often have a very low intake of this nutrient.

The two most widely ingested forms of omega-3 fatty acids, docosahexaenoic acid (DHA) and eicosapentaenoic acid (EPA), derive primarily from fish oil. They have a powerful protective effect on our cardiovascular system, immune system, brain, bones, muscles, joints, lungs, liver, skin, hair, and eyes, among many other body tissues.

Another important omega-3 fatty acid is the famous alpha-linolenic acid (ALA), which comes from plant sources such as flaxseed oil, canola oil, nuts, and some fruits. However, it possesses only a fraction of the benefits of DHA and EPA.

It is advisable that you consume between 400 and 500 milligrams of DHA or EPA per week to be in good health, but if you are an athlete or train intensely, you should consume between 3 and 4 grams daily, preferably spread over 3 to 4 doses of one gram each.

## CONCLUSION

Always remember that the key to intelligent supplementation is to individualize your requirements, and that is only possible by going to a qualified specialist who can guide you on what is best for you. Don't experiment with your health.

# 10.

# FREQUENTLY ASKED QUESTIONS

**M**any women and girls write to me every day through social media. Everyone wants to know things about my personal life, my food, my routines. They even ask me about how I manage to resist the temptations of sweets and parties. I don't think I have all the answers; I don't even think I'm always doing the right thing. I do what works for me, and if I'm wrong, I fall, or I'm stuck, I try to change as fast as possible, without regrets. It's normal to fall. What's bad is if you stay crying on the floor and don't get up.

We have selected some frequently asked questions. If yours is here, I think you'll have my most honest answer. But always remember, my advice works only if you apply it to your own life with motivation and discipline. Just reading this won't make you strong. The dumbbells will.

### Do fruits help you lose weight?

Yes, provided that you consume them in the right quantity and quality. Why? Fruits are rich in natural sugars, but they are also loaded with fiber that keeps the sugar "locked in," causing it to be digested and passed to the blood more slowly. Fruits are a good choice to satisfy sweet cravings, and they also improve your digestive functioning. Fruit sugar doesn't accumulate as fat as easily as table sugar or the sugar found in white bread. If you want to lose weight and lower your body-fat percentage, the most recommended fruits are kiwi, peach, orange, tangerine, strawberry, green apple, blackberry, passion fruit, grapefruit, blueberries, cherries, melon, pineapple, tamarind, and lemon. Try to eat them before training to have an energy boost, or eat them in the morning.

### When it comes to losing weight, what works best: food or exercise?

BOTH OF THEM! It is all or nothing. If you eat healthily and choose the right foods 90 percent of the time and you maintain an adequate exercise routine, I promise you will see results. Now, if you eat poorly all day, I promise you'll be wasting your time at the gym. You will spend hours upon hours and you will not see any progress. I'll explain it in a practical way: if you drop 500 or 700 calories a day from your diet during a week, you'll be saving 4,900 calories a week. If you exercise (one hour of cardio and 30 to 40 minutes of weights) five days a week you can burn between 500 and 800 calories per day, and in a week you will be burning some 2,500 to 4,000 extra calories. The sum is perfect! With 4,900 calories saved from healthy eating and at least 2,500 calories burned while exercising, the total is 7,400 calories. That's like losing a kilogram of fat per week!

### Can I add all the olive oil I want to a salad, since it's considered a good fat?

Definitely not! Remember when I told you about that stagnation that I myself experienced? Well, I learned that everything in excess causes fat gain. We all know that olive oil is famous for its benefits, but although it is indeed super healthy, in excess it will make you gain weight. Olive oil provides nine calories per gram, so a teaspoon provides forty-five calories. That's the amount that should be consumed at each meal.

### Can I replace food with protein powder in order to lose weight?

High-quality whey protein is a good choice because it is nutritious, easily absorbed by the body, and very easy to prepare and transport, especially when you have little time and you're running around. It's difficult to carry a chicken breast or a piece of salmon in your bag all the time. However, the healthiest option is to use it as a food supplement and not a meal replacement. Your body needs to chew, taste, and eat for real. That's why the secret is to organize and plan your meals ahead of time.

### If I replace the amount of processed sugar I eat with the equivalent amount in natural sugar, will my fat levels be affected?

Sources of natural sugar (fruits, grains, tubers, and so on) have fiber in addition to sugar. As I explained above, fiber keeps the sugar "enclosed," which means it doesn't accumulate as fat so quickly. Processed sugar is a different story altogether, because it is easily digested and quickly absorbed. It quickly passes into the bloodstream, and your body turns it into fat almost immediately.

But beware! If you consume too much natural sugar, or more natural sugar than your body needs, the fiber won't be able to "catch it all," and your body will also store it as fat. I told you before and I'll tell you again: everything in excess is fattening. Period.

### Is red meat a bad source of protein?

Red meat is an excellent source of protein, but unlike white meat, it contains more saturated fats, which, if consumed in excess, can be harmful to the heart and colon, in addition to the fact that it provides your body with many more calories. It is best to consume red meats no more than twice a week, but you don't need to eliminate them entirely. When consuming red meats, favor leaner cuts, for example beef tenderloin. Remove as much fat as possible before cooking, and remove the melted fat after cooking. Bake it or grill it, and accompany it with plenty of vegetables. Avoid eating processed meats—such as bacon, mortadella, salami, and sausages, among others—at all costs. All of these are high in fat and sodium, making it difficult for you to get toned or lose weight.

### Is red wine fattening?

Everything in excess is fattening—remember? I don't want to sound like a broken record, but yes. Each gram of alcohol contains seven calories, regardless of the drink. That is, all alcoholic beverages, in excess, will cause you to gain weight. But actually, the main problem with calories derived from alcohol is that they do not contribute any nutrients—they are "empty calories." Our body does not use them; it simply stores them as fat. If you want to achieve a toned body and lower your fat percentage, avoid alcoholic beverages, or consume them only occasionally. There is no result without sacrifice.

### Are diet sodas pure poison?

Drinking a reasonable amount of diet soda occasionally, like a can here and there, won't hurt you. The artificial sweeteners and other chemicals currently used in diet sodas are safe and there is no serious evidence that these ingredients cause cancer. But I want to make it clear that diet sodas are not the healthiest choice or solution for weight loss. Although switching from regular soda to diet soda can save you calories, it can also stimulate cravings for sweets. There are better options, such as natural water, sugar-free flavored water, and teas and floral infusions. The latter provide antioxidants and aren't full of harmful chemicals like soda.

### Is the best way to lose fat not eating fat at all?

The best way to lose fat is to get off the couch and exercise. There is no other way. Your body requires a daily amount of nutrients, and if you exceed the amount you need, or if you don't burn what you eat because you're sitting all the time, you store the excess calories in the form of fat. Yes, excess fat, as well as excess proteins and carbohydrates, accumulates in the body and is "stored" as fat. So it's time to change what you think and get moving to get the results you expect.

### I stopped doing cheat meals because I gained weight thirty minutes after each one. Why does that happen?

Cheat meals are good metabolism accelerators. Giving your body something it was not expecting is like adding coal to the fire. The body will feel rewarded, it will believe that the time has come not to have to hold on to its fat reserves, and it will start to burn much more. It's something that is perfectly accepted by our body, both mentally and physically. In addition, cheat meals prevent you from falling into the temptation to leave the diet, as you could think of them as a motivator of sorts, since you know that on a certain day you can enjoy all the food you want, and then continue to eat right during the rest of the week.

Now, most of the foods we crave are loaded with fats and salt, so you will probably feel a little bloated or heavy after eating them. But that effect is momentary, and you will lose it as soon as you start following your meal plan again.

### If I eat too much protein, will it turn into fat?

Just like carbohydrates and fats, proteins provide calories. In fact, one gram of protein has exactly the same amount of calories as one gram of carbohydrate (four kilocalories). When you eat too many proteins, your body cannot store them as proteins so it turns them into carbohydrates or fats—exactly what you don't want, right? Many believe that it is better to eat more proteins, but each person is different! I recommend that you consult with your nutritionist to find out what the right amount is for you.

### Is it okay to eat carbs after noon?

Carbohydrates are fuel for your body, and it's impossible to sustain an intense effort like exercising for a prolonged amount of time without the correct amount of energy. But it all depends on the quality and quantity of the exercise you do.

Fiber-rich sources of carbohydrates such as vegetables and grains provide energy that lasts up to six hours after you consume them. If you train at night, you can eat your fiber-rich carbohydrates at lunchtime in order to maintain high energy levels for a good workout. Or if you train very early in the morning, you can eat them at night in order to increase your energy reserve. But beware of refined carbohydrates such as those found in table sugar, pastries, and refined flour, which don't provide energy for long periods of time and therefore make it difficult to lose fat.

### Is it bad to have a low body-fat percentage?

Your body's fat percentage needs to be kept at the proper level for it to continue to function. Fat acts as the body's insulator, and thanks to it you can regulate your body temperature and carry vitamins in the body. Having too low a body-fat percentage could cause serious problems. Additionally, fat is an important part of the body structure. It helps the functioning of the nervous system and even constitutes certain hormones, including those that support fertility. One of the potential consequences of having a low body-fat percentage is that women cease to have their menstrual periods, which completely changes the inner working of the female body. A little body fat isn't bad, and in fact it also contours your body and works as a protection pad for many organs.

### Is stevia the healthiest and most natural sweetener?

Stevia is a calorie-free plant with sweetening properties. It is much healthier than saccharin, aspartame, cyclamate, thaumatin, and sucralose, which are also zero-calorie sweeteners, but with artificial ingredients which can affect your cravings for sweets and, in some cases, your health. I always prefer the most natural option: stevia.

### Should I fast or should I eat before exercising?

The answer is: both! Whether or not you should eat before your training session depends on several factors. First, some people simply prefer not to eat because their stomachs cannot tolerate exercising while full—they often feel discomfort or nausea. Others prefer not to eat before exercising in order to burn more fat. When the body is fasting, it mobilizes and burns stored fats, but whether or not your body uses those fat reserves as energy will depend on your level of training. In people with a high level of training, the body is able to use that fat as energy. But in the case of people who are just starting to exercise and people who aren't in very good shape, their bodies mobilize those fats but, instead of burning them, cling on to them. In other words, they waste all their hard work! If you belong to this group of people, it's best to eat something before exercising, because it will help increase your calorie burn and prevent you from destroying your muscles in order to produce energy. However, it will also depend on the type of exercise you are going to do and how long you are going to do it. The body has energy reserves for an hour of exercise in the form of carbohydrates and virtually unlimited reserves of fat. If you prefer to exercise on an empty stomach, choose exercises of moderate intensity that do not exceed an hour. If you are one of those people who cannot tolerate food before exercising, or you find it difficult to exercise with a full stomach, I think it is best not to have breakfast—but make sure you hydrate very well, and you can eat a fruit and follow the same indications I just mentioned above. As soon as you finish your training session, eat a balanced breakfast to replenish your energy reserves and recover quickly.

# CONCLUSION

**Y**ou have what you need. Now it's time to act. . . .

If you read this book carefully, I think you will have learned many new things. I also hope you have been able to learn from my mistakes and successes—that's exactly why I wrote this book. Now you know my nutrition, supplementation, and training secrets. That's very good news. The bad news is that everything you learned here will do you no good if you don't close this book, find the best motivation within you, and begin to apply my eating tips and go running to do your routines, every day.

Never forget that the Hot Body Diet is a twenty-eight-day diet plan that will help you overcome your own barriers and achieve your best self in a fabulous, strong, and healthy body. And you can repeat this plan as many times as you need. The greatest result you will ever get is that you will gain joy, self-esteem, and energy.

Dr. Samar Yorde and I have shown you the secrets of food, the importance of taking the right supplements, and how to accelerate your metabolism so that your body becomes a fat-burning machine all the time. We also made easy and tasty recipes so you can enjoy the process and not get bored along the way.

Now that you know what to do and how to do it, what is your excuse?

It all comes down to eating right, exercising your machine, supplementing it correctly, getting enough rest, and overcoming anxiety. You know that your mind is your worst enemy, because therein lies the root of your weight gain, your frustrations, and your laziness. That's why you must attack them with your mind. Your first battle against fat takes place in your mind. If you change your way of thinking, you find a great passion, and you do what you have to do, no one will be able to keep up.

You already have the power of knowledge. Now you just have to start. Just like that. Get out of the chair you're sitting in, get out of bed, go shop for what you need. Let's go, girl. Go find your clothes, your food, and your hydration and start now. Once you enter this world and see the changes in your body and mind, you will never want to stop.

Do you want to be fabulous and confident and look spectacular at any age? Never waste time again complaining, eating in front of the TV, and criticizing women who look beautiful in their dresses or bathing suits. Never buy that extra-large-sized dress again in order to hide your body. Stop hiding behind fat and excuses, and move your ass right now!

I once read a fable about a gazelle and a lion. Every morning in Africa, a gazelle wakes up. She knows that she has to run faster than the lion or he will eat her. And every morning in Africa, a lion awakes as well. He knows he must be faster than the slowest gazelle or he will starve. It doesn't matter whether you're a lion or a gazelle: when the new day arrives you'd better be running.

Life is like a lion. And we are all born gazelles. If you don't run, if you don't act, life will eat you up. Time passes and so do opportunities. I want you to be a lioness. Don't let life pass you by. You're the one who needs to make your way through life leaving traces, firm and indelible, in your work, your home, your environment, but above all in yourself. I hope you are determined to become a lioness, because I stopped being a gazelle long ago.

Don't sit around waiting for your next life. You have the beauty you need. All you need is to polish it and show it to the world. Today, start treating yourself with love and respect. Be mindful of what you feed your body, what you put into your mind, and what you decide every day. Your results will be the consequence of every little decision you make every day.

Enjoy the sun, energy, joy, self-love, partner, and good life you will have when you start to burn fat, tone your muscles, and build that body that will make all men stare at you like fools. Start enjoying it now. Visualize yourself, beautiful and secure, walking past those who have criticized you over time. Prove to yourself that you will go as far as you decide to go. Your beauty, your fitness, and your joy will open all doors.

Fall in love with your life, eat healthily, think right, and do your best. Happiness is in your self-esteem and the confidence you have in yourself.

Remember that your body is made to burn fat—you just have to use it, so turn it on daily. To stay active I encourage you to download my workouts at https://www.fitplanapp.com/athletes/michelle-lewin, or start training with my platform at www.lewinfitnessplatform.com, right now.

I invite you to stay connected through my social media accounts, my YouTube channel, and my website, www.michellelewin.com, where you can find my monthly calendar of events and information on where I'm going to be. It would be great to be able to meet you at one of those events; I'd love for you to tell me about your experience and your results with this book.

Write to me through social media—@michelle_lewin on Instagram and Twitter, and Michelle Lewin on Facebook and YouTube—and show me how your body and your mind have changed since you've read my words. I want to see you succeed.

Do your thing!

Michelle Lewin

# WORKS CITED

1.  Circo F. *Actividad física y ejercicio físico: Las diferencias entre ambos términos*. Available at: http://www.instructorado-iafa.com.ar/articulos/ejercicio-actividad-fisica.pdf.

2.  *Organización Mundial de la Salud 10 causas principales de defunción. Actualizado en 2008*. Available at: http://www.who.int/mediacentre/factsheets/fs310/es/index.html.

3.  American College of Sports Medicine. *ACSM's Guidelines for Exercise Testing and Prescription*. Philadelphia: Lippincott, Williams & Wilkins, 2002.

4.  Bray, G. *Office Management of Obesity*, 2nd ed. 2004.

5.  Bastien M, Poirier P, Lemieux I, Després JP. "Overview of Epidemiology and Contribution of Obesity to Cardiovascular Disease." *Progress in Cardiovascular Diseases*. January–February 2014, 56(4): 369–81.

6.  World Health Organization (WHO). "Physical Status: The Use and Interpretation of Anthropometry: A Report of a WHO Expert Committee." Technical Report Series. Rome: 1995, 854: 1–452.

7.  National Physique Committee. "NPC Bikini Division Rules." Available at: http://npcnewsonline.com/npc-bikini-division-rules/.

8.  Li WC, Chen IC, Chang YC, Loke SS, Wang SH, Hsiao KY. "Waist-to-Height Ratio, Waist Circumference, and Body Mass Index as Indices of Cardiometabolic Risk Among 36,642 Taiwanese Adults." *European Journal of Nutrition*. 2013 Feb, 52(1): 57–65.

9.  Lim SS, Vos T, Flaxman AD, Danaei G, Shibuya K, Adair-Rohani H et al. "A Comparative Risk Assessment of Burden of Disease and Injury Attributable to 67 Risk Factors and Risk Factor Clusters in 21 Regions, 1990–2010: A Systematic Analysis for the Global Burden of Disease Study (2010)." *Lancet*. 2012, 380(9859): 2224–60.

10. Berning JM, Adams KJ, Stamford BA. "Anabolic Steroid Usage in Athletics: Facts, Fiction, and Public Relations." *The Journal of Strength & Conditioning Research*. 2004, 18(4): 908–17.

11. Blair SN, Kohl HW, Gordon BF, Paffenbarger RS. "How Much Physical Activity Is Good for Health?" *Annual Review of Public Health*. 1992, 13: 99–126.

12. Kiningham RB, Apgar BS, Schwenk TL. "Evaluation of Amenorrhea." *American Family Physician Journal*. 1996, 53: 1185–1194.

13. American College of Sports Medicine. "ACSM's Quantity and Quality of Exercise for Developing and Maintaining Cardiorespiratory, Musculoskeletal, and Neuromotor Fitness in Apparently Healthy Adults: Guidance for Prescribing Exercise." July 2011, 43(7): 1334–59.

14. American Heart Association. "Know Your Fats (2010)." Available at: http://www.heart.org/HEARTORG/Conditions/Cholesterol/PreventionTreatmentofHighCholesterol/Know-Your-Fats_UCM_305628_Article.jsp.

15. *Organización Mundial de la salud. "Estrategia mundial sobre régimen alimentario, actividad física y salud"* (2004). Available at: http://www.who.int/dietphysicalactivity/strategy/eb11344/strategy_spanish_web.pdf.

16. Medical Institute. *Sleep Disorders and Sleep Deprivation: An Unmet Public Health Problem*. Washington, DC: The National Academies Press, 2006.

17. Position of the American Dietetic Association, Dietitians of Canada, and the American College of Sports Medicine. "Nutrition and Athletic Performance." *Journal of the American Dietetic Association*. 2000, 39(12): 1543–56.

18. Ramsay TG. "Fat Cells." *Endocrinology and Metabolism Clinics of North America*. December 1996, 25(4): 847–70.

19. Guyton, A. *Tratado de Fisiología Médica*, 11th ed. Madrid: Elsevier España, 2006.

20. Berning J., Nelson Oteen S. *Nutrition for Sport & Exercise*, 2nd ed. Gaithersburg: Aspen Publishers, 1998.

21. Instituto nacional sobre el envejecimiento. *"Ejercicio y Actividad Física: Su guía diaria."* Washington, DC, publication no. 10-4931s, 2010.

22. Fernández Vaquero A. *"Respuesta cardíaca al ejercicio."* In: López Chicharro J, Fernández Vaquero A, editores. *Fisiología del Ejercicio*, 3rd ed. Madrid: Ed. Panamericana, 2006.

23. Association AD. *"Edulcorantes Artificiales,"* 2013, cited 13 February 2017. Available from: http://www.diabetes.org/espanol/nutricion-y-recetas/edulcorantes-artificiales/.

24. Ruiz-Roso B, Pérez-Olleros L, García-Cuevas M. *"Influencia de la fibra dietaria (FD) en la biodisponibilidad de los nutrientes"* (2001) In: *Fibra Dietética en Iberoamérica: Tecnología y salud: Obtención, caracterización, efecto fisiológico y aplicación en alimentos*. São Paulo, Brazil: Varela Editora e Libraría LTDA, 2001, 345–70.

25. García-Arias, MT, García-Fernández, MC. *Nutrición y Dietética*. Editorial Universidad de León, 2003.

26. Hinton P, Sanford T, Davidson MM, Yakushko O, Beck N. "Nutrient Intake and Dietary Behaviors of Male and Female Collegiate Athletes." *International Journal of Sports Nutrition and Exercise Metabolism*. 2004, 14(4): 389–90.

27. Boyer J, Liu R. "Apple Phytochemicals and Their Health Benefits." *Nutrition Journal.* May 12, 2004, 3: 5.

28. Jimeno, A, Ballesteros, M, Ugedo, L. *Biología.* Fuenlabrada: Santillana, 1997.

29. American College of Sports Medicine, American Dietetic Association, and Dietitians of Canada. "Joint Position Statement: Nutrition and Athletic Performance." *Medicine & Science in Sports & Exercise.* 2000, 32: 2130–45.

30. American Heart Association. "Eat More Chicken, Fish and Beans Than Red Meat" (2013). Available in: http://www.heart.org/HEARTORG/GettingHealthy/WeightManagement/LosingWeight/Eat-More-Chicken-Fish-and-Beans-than-Red-Meat_UCM_320278_Article.jsp.

31. Organización Mundial de la Salud. *"Estrategia mundial sobre régimen alimentario: Fomento del consumo mundial de frutas y verduras"* (2013). Available at: http://www.who.int/dietphysicalactivity/fruit/es/index1.html.

32. Castro-Rodríguez, Martinez-Fernandez, Perote-Alejandre. Instituto Tomás Pascual Sanz. *"Vive Sano,"* (2012). Available at: www.institutotomaspascual.es.

33. American Heart Association. "AHA Recommendation: Milk Products" (2013). Available at: http://www.heart.org/HEARTORG/GettingHealthy/NutritionCenter/Milk-Products_UCM_306008_Article.jsp.

34. Marcason W. "How Many Grams of Trans-Fat Are Recommended per Day?" *Journal of the American Dietetic Association.* September 2006, 106(9): 1507.

35. *Instituto del Corazón de Texas. "Vitaminas: cómo actúan y dónde conseguirlas"* (2013). Available at: http://www.texasheartinstitute.org/HIC/Topics_Esp/HSmart/vita_sp.cfm.

36. National Institutes of Health, Office of Dietary Supplements. *"Información para el consumidor."* Available at: http://ods.od.nih.gov/HealthInformation/RecursosEnEspanol.aspx.

37. Costill, DL, Sparks, KE. "Rapid Fluid Replacement Following Dehydration." *Journal of Applied Physiology,* 1973, 34: 36–43.

38. Adolph, EF. "Blood Changes in Dehydration." In: Adolph, EF, ed. *Physiology of Man in the Desert.* New York: Interscience, 1947, 160–71.

39. Olveira-Fuster G, Gonzalo-Marín M. (2007). *"Actualización en requerimientos nutricionales." Endocrinología y Nutrición.* 2007, 54(supl 2): 17–29.

40. Campbell N, Correa-Rotter R, Neal B, Cappuccio FP. "New Evidence Relating to the Health Impact of Reducing Salt Intake." *Nutrition, Metabolism and Cardiovascular Diseases.* 2001, 21: 617–19.

41. Ortega RM, López-Sobaler AM, Ballesteros JM, Pérez-Farinós N, Rodríguez- Rodríguez E, Aparicio A, Perea JM, Andrés P. (2011). "Estimation of Salt Intake by 24 H Urinary Sodium Excretion in a Representative Sample of Spanish Adults." *British Journal of Nutrition.* 2011, 105: 787–94.

42. Centers for Disease Control and Prevention. National Center for Chronic Disease Prevention and Health Promotion, Office on Smoking and Health,

Department of Health and Human Services. "Smoking and Tobacco Use—Fact Sheet: Health Effects of Cigarette Smoking." Updated January 2008. Available at: http://www.cdc.gov/tobacco/data_statistics/fact_sheets/health_effects/effects_cig_smoking/index.htm.

43. World Health Organization. "Diet, Nutrition and the Prevention of Chronic Diseases. Report of a Joint WHO/FAO Expert Consultation." Technical Report Series. Rome: 2003, 916.

44. US Food and Drug Administration. "Food Label Helps Consumers Make Healthier Choices." Available at: www.fda.gov/downloads/forconsumers/consumerupdates/ucm199361.pdf.

45. Vieira, G. "Do You Have a Cheat Meal?" Available at: http://www.diabetesdaily.com/blog/2012/07/do-you-have-a-cheat-meal.

46. Ruiz, J. *"Nutrición."* Available at: www.jruizl.es.

47. Kreider RB, Wilborn CD, Taylor L, Campbell B, Almada AL, Collins R et al. "ISSN Exercise & Sport Nutrition Review: Research & Recommendations." *Journal of the International Society of Sports Nutrition.* 2010 7: 1–35.

48. Maughan RJ, Depiesse F, Geyer H. "The Use of Dietary Supplements by Athletes." *Journal of Sports Sciences,* 2007.

49. Campbell et al. "International Society of Sports Nutrition Position Stand: Protein and Exercise." *Journal of the International Society of Sports Nutrition,* 2007.

50. Tipton KD, Wolfe RR. "Protein and Amino Acids for Athletes." *Journal of Sports Sciences,* 2004.

51. Garlick PJ. "The Role of Leucine in the Regulation of Protein Metabolism." *Journal of Nutrition,* 2005.

52. Koopman R, Verdijk L, Manders RFJ, Gijsen AP, Gorselink M, Pijpers E et al. "Co-ingestion of Protein and Leucine Stimulates Muscle Protein Synthesis Rates to the Same Extent in Young and Elderly Lean Men." *The American Journal of Clinical Nutrition,* 2006.

53. Baptista IL, Leal ML, Artioli GG, Aoki MS, Fiamoncini J, Turri AO et al. "Leucine Attenuates Skeletal Muscle Wasting via Inhibition of Ubiquitin Ligases." *Muscle Nerve,* 2010.

54. Laviano A, Muscaritoli M, Cascino A, Preziosa I, Inui A, Mantovani G et al. "Branched-chain Amino Acids: The Best Compromise to Achieve Anabolism?" *Current Opinion in Clinical Nutrition & Metabolic Care.* 2005, 8: 408–14.

55. Buford et al. "International Society of Sport Nutrition Position Stand: Creatine Supplementation and Exercise." *Journal of the International Society of Sports Nutrition,* 2007.

56. Kim et al. "Studies on the Safety of Creatine Supplementation." *Amino Acids,* 2011.

57. Goldstein et al. "International Society of Sports Nutrition Position Stand: Caffeine and Performance." *Journal of the International Society of Sports Nututrition,* 2010.

58.   Shixian et al. "Green Tea Extract Thermogenesis-induced Weight Loss by Epigallocatechin Gallate Inhibition of Catechol-O-methyltransferase." *Journal of Medicinal Food*, 2006.

59.   Sawka et al. "Exercise and Fluid Replacement." American College of Sports Medicine, 2007.

60.   Snell PG, Ward R, Kandaswami C, Stohs SJ. "Comparative Effects of Selected Non-caffeinated Rehydration Sports Drinks on Short-term Performance Following Moderate Dehydration." *Journal of the International Society of Sports Nutrition*, 2010.

61.   Machefer G, Groussard C, Zouhal H, Vincent S, Youssef H, Faure H et al. "Nutritional and Plasmatic Antioxidant Vitamins Status of Ultra-endurance Athletes." *The Journal of the American College of Nutrition*, 2007.

62.   Bailey RL, Fulgoni III VL, Keast DR, Dwyer JT. "Examination of Vitamin Intake Among US Adults Using Dietary Supplements." *Journal of the Academy of Nutrition and Dietetics*, 2012.

63.   Li, D. "Chemistry Behind Vegetarianism." *Journal of Agriculture and Food Chemistry*, 2011.

64.   Calder PC, Deckelbaum RJ. "Omega-3 Fatty Acids: Time to Get the Message Right!" *Current Opinion in Clinical Nutrition & Metabolic Care*, 2008.

65.   Wang C, Harris WS, Chung W, Lichtenstein AH, Balk EM, Kupelnick B et al. "N-3 Fatty Acids from Fish or Fish-oil Supplements, but Not α-linolenic Acid, Benefit Cardiovascular Disease Outcomes in Primary- and Secondary-prevention Studies: A Systematic Review." *The American Journal of Clinical Nutrition*, 2006.

66.   Davis M. "Broad Spectrum Cardiac Protection with Fish Oil." *Life Extension*, September 2006.

67.   Mazza M, Pomponi M, Janiri L, Brai P, Mazza S. "Omega-3 Fatty Acids and Antioxidants in Neurological and Psychiatric Diseases: An Overview." *Progress in Neuro-Psychopharmacology & Biological Psychiatry*, 2007.

68.   Novak F, Heyland DK, Avenell A, Drover JW, Su X. "Glutamine Supplementation in Serious Illness: A Systematic Review of the Evidence." *Critical Care Medicine*, 2002.

69.   Burrin DG, Stoll B. "Metabolic Fate and Function of Dietary Glutamate in the Gut." *The American Journal of Clinical Nutrition*, 2009.

70.   Zhou M, Martindale RG. "Arginine in the Critical Care Setting." *Journal of Nutrition*, 2007.

71.   Buijs N, van Brokhorst-de van der Schueren MAE, Languis JAE, Leemans CR, Kuik DJ, Vermeulen MA et al. "Perioperative Arginine-supplemented Nutrition in Malnourished Patients with Head and Neck Cancer Improves Long-term Survival." *The American Journal of Clinical Nutrition*, 2011.

# appendices

# FOOD AND SUPPLEMENT CHECKLIST

## WEEK 1

| TIME | FOOD/SUPPLEMENTS | DAY 1 | DAY 2 | DAY 3 | DAY 4 | DAY 5 | DAY 6 | DAY 7 |
|---|---|---|---|---|---|---|---|---|
| 6 A.M. TO 7 A.M. | MEAL 1: PRE-WORKOUT SNACK | | | | | | | |
| | SUPPLEMENTS | | | | | | | |
| | | | | | | | | |
| | | | | | | | | |
| | | | | | | | | |
| | | | | | | | | |
| | | | | | | | | |
| 8 A.M. TO 9 A.M. | MEAL 2: BREAKFAST | | | | | | | |
| | SUPPLEMENTS | | | | | | | |
| | | | | | | | | |
| | | | | | | | | |
| | | | | | | | | |
| | | | | | | | | |
| | | | | | | | | |
| 12 P.M. TO 1 P.M. | MEAL 3: LUNCH | | | | | | | |
| | SUPPLEMENTS | | | | | | | |
| | | | | | | | | |
| | | | | | | | | |
| 3 P.M. TO 4 P.M. | MEAL 4: SNACK P.M. 1 | | | | | | | |
| | SUPPLEMENTS | | | | | | | |
| | | | | | | | | |
| 6 P.M. TO 7 P.M. | MEAL 5: DINNER | | | | | | | |
| | SUPPLEMENTS | | | | | | | |
| | | | | | | | | |
| 9 P.M. TO 10 P.M. | MEAL 6: SNACK P.M. 2 | | | | | | | |
| | SUPPLEMENTS | | | | | | | |
| | | | | | | | | |
| | | | | | | | | |

# WEEK 2

| TIME | FOOD/SUPPLEMENTS | DAY 8 | DAY 9 | DAY 10 | DAY 11 | DAY 12 | DAY 13 | DAY 14 |
|---|---|---|---|---|---|---|---|---|
| **6 A.M. TO 7 A.M.** | MEAL 1: PRE-WORKOUT SNACK | | | | | | | |
| | SUPPLEMENTS | | | | | | | |
| | | | | | | | | |
| | | | | | | | | |
| | | | | | | | | |
| | | | | | | | | |
| | | | | | | | | |
| **8 A.M. TO 9 A.M.** | MEAL 2: BREAKFAST | | | | | | | |
| | SUPPLEMENTS | | | | | | | |
| | | | | | | | | |
| | | | | | | | | |
| | | | | | | | | |
| | | | | | | | | |
| | | | | | | | | |
| **12 P.M. TO 1 P.M.** | MEAL 3: LUNCH | | | | | | | |
| | SUPPLEMENTS | | | | | | | |
| | | | | | | | | |
| | | | | | | | | |
| **3 P.M. TO 4 P.M.** | MEAL 4: SNACK P.M. 1 | | | | | | | |
| | SUPPLEMENTS | | | | | | | |
| | | | | | | | | |
| **6 P.M. TO 7 P.M.** | MEAL 5: DINNER | | | | | | | |
| | SUPPLEMENTS | | | | | | | |
| | | | | | | | | |
| **9 P.M. TO 10 P.M.** | MEAL 6: SNACK P.M. 2 | | | | | | | |
| | SUPPLEMENTS | | | | | | | |
| | | | | | | | | |
| | | | | | | | | |

# WEEK 3

| TIME | FOOD/SUPPLEMENTS | DAY 15 | DAY 16 | DAY 17 | DAY 18 | DAY 19 | DAY 20 | DAY 21 |
|---|---|---|---|---|---|---|---|---|
| **6 A.M. TO 7 A.M.** | MEAL 1: PRE-WORKOUT SNACK | | | | | | | |
| | SUPPLEMENTS | | | | | | | |
| | | | | | | | | |
| | | | | | | | | |
| | | | | | | | | |
| | | | | | | | | |
| | | | | | | | | |
| **8 A.M. TO 9 A.M.** | MEAL 2: BREAKFAST | | | | | | | |
| | SUPPLEMENTS | | | | | | | |
| | | | | | | | | |
| | | | | | | | | |
| | | | | | | | | |
| | | | | | | | | |
| | | | | | | | | |
| **12 P.M. TO 1 P.M.** | MEAL 3: LUNCH | | | | | | | |
| | SUPPLEMENTS | | | | | | | |
| | | | | | | | | |
| | | | | | | | | |
| **3 P.M. TO 4 P.M.** | MEAL 4: SNACK P.M. 1 | | | | | | | |
| | SUPPLEMENTS | | | | | | | |
| | | | | | | | | |
| **6 P.M. TO 7 P.M.** | MEAL 5: DINNER | | | | | | | |
| | SUPPLEMENTS | | | | | | | |
| | | | | | | | | |
| **9 P.M. TO 10 P.M.** | MEAL 6: SNACK P.M. 2 | | | | | | | |
| | SUPPLEMENTS | | | | | | | |
| | | | | | | | | |
| | | | | | | | | |

## WEEK 4

| TIME | FOOD/SUPPLEMENTS | DAY 22 | DAY 23 | DAY 24 | DAY 25 | DAY 26 | DAY 27 | DAY 28 |
|------|------------------|--------|--------|--------|--------|--------|--------|--------|
| 6 A.M. TO 7 A.M. | MEAL 1: PRE-WORKOUT SNACK | | | | | | | |
| | SUPPLEMENTS | | | | | | | |
| | | | | | | | | |
| | | | | | | | | |
| | | | | | | | | |
| | | | | | | | | |
| | | | | | | | | |
| 8 A.M. TO 9 A.M. | MEAL 2: BREAKFAST | | | | | | | |
| | SUPPLEMENTS | | | | | | | |
| | | | | | | | | |
| | | | | | | | | |
| | | | | | | | | |
| | | | | | | | | |
| | | | | | | | | |
| 12 P.M. TO 1 P.M. | MEAL 3: LUNCH | | | | | | | |
| | SUPPLEMENTS | | | | | | | |
| | | | | | | | | |
| | | | | | | | | |
| 3 P.M. TO 4 P.M. | MEAL 4: SNACK P.M. 1 | | | | | | | |
| | SUPPLEMENTS | | | | | | | |
| | | | | | | | | |
| 6 P.M. TO 7 P.M. | MEAL 5: DINNER | | | | | | | |
| | SUPPLEMENTS | | | | | | | |
| | | | | | | | | |
| 9 P.M. TO 10 P.M. | MEAL 6: SNACK P.M. 2 | | | | | | | |
| | SUPPLEMENTS | | | | | | | |
| | | | | | | | | |
| | | | | | | | | |

APPENDICES: FOOD AND SUPPLEMENT CHECKLIST

# EXERCISE CHECKLIST

## WEEK 1

| EXERCISE | DAY 1 | DAY 2 | DAY 3 | DAY 4 | DAY 5 | DAY 6 | DAY 7 |
|---|---|---|---|---|---|---|---|
| CARDIO<br>30 to 45 minutes, 6 times a week<br>Power walking, running, cycling, stair-climbing, jumping rope, spinning, kickboxing, skating, rowing, dancing, skiing, swimming, elliptical | | | | | | | |
| HIGH-INTENSITY INTERVAL TRAINING (HIIT)<br>3 times a week | | | | | | | |
| LOW-INTENSITY STEADY-STATE TRAINING (LISS)<br>3 times a week | | | | | | | |
| STRENGTH<br>5 times a week<br>3 exercises—4 series of 20, 15, 12, and 10 repetitions<br>One day per group<br>Glutes—quadriceps—femorals—biceps/triceps—shoulders/back | | | | | | | |
| ABDOMINALS<br>3 days a week<br>3 exercises—4 series of 25 repetitions | | | | | | | |

Download https://www.fitplanapp.com/athletes/michelle-lewin, or train with my platform: www.lewinfitnessplatform.com.

# WEEK 2

| EXERCISE | DAY 8 | DAY 9 | DAY 10 | DAY 11 | DAY 12 | DAY 13 | DAY 14 |
|---|---|---|---|---|---|---|---|
| CARDIO<br>30 to 45 minutes, 6 times a week<br>Power walking, running, cycling, stair-climbing, jumping rope, spinning, kickboxing, skating, rowing, dancing, skiing, swimming, elliptical | | | | | | | |
| HIGH-INTENSITY INTERVAL TRAINING (HIIT)<br>3 times a week | | | | | | | |
| LOW-INTENSITY STEADY-STATE TRAINING (LISS)<br>3 times a week | | | | | | | |
| STRENGTH<br>5 times a week<br>3 exercises—4 series of 20, 15, 12, and 10 repetitions<br>One day per group<br>Glutes—quadriceps—femorals—biceps/triceps—shoulders/back | | | | | | | |
| ABDOMINALS<br>3 days a week<br>3 exercises—4 series of 25 repetitions | | | | | | | |

Download https://www.fitplanapp.com/athletes/michelle-lewin, or train with my platform: www.lewinfitnessplatform.com.

# WEEK 3

| EXERCISE | DAY 15 | DAY 16 | DAY 17 | DAY 18 | DAY 19 | DAY 20 | DAY 21 |
|---|---|---|---|---|---|---|---|
| CARDIO<br>30 to 45 minutes, 6 times a week<br>Power walking, running, cycling, stair-climbing, jumping rope, spinning, kickboxing, skating, rowing, dancing, skiing, swimming, elliptical | | | | | | | |
| HIGH-INTENSITY INTERVAL TRAINING (HIIT)<br>3 times a week | | | | | | | |
| LOW-INTENSITY STEADY-STATE TRAINING (LISS)<br>3 times a week | | | | | | | |
| STRENGTH<br>5 times a week<br>3 exercises—4 series of 20, 15, 12, and 10 repetitions<br>One day per group<br>Glutes—quadriceps—femorals—biceps/triceps—shoulders/back | | | | | | | |
| ABDOMINALS<br>3 days a week<br>3 exercises—4 series of 25 repetitions | | | | | | | |

Download https://www.fitplanapp.com/athletes/michelle-lewin, or train with my platform: www.lewinfitnessplatform.com.

# WEEK 4

| EXERCISE | DAY 22 | DAY 23 | DAY 24 | DAY 25 | DAY 26 | DAY 27 | DAY 28 |
|---|---|---|---|---|---|---|---|
| CARDIO<br>30 to 45 minutes, 6 times a week<br>Power walking, running, cycling, stair-climbing, jumping rope, spinning, kickboxing, skating, rowing, dancing, skiing, swimming, elliptical | | | | | | | |
| HIGH-INTENSITY INTERVAL TRAINING (HIIT)<br>3 times a week | | | | | | | |
| LOW-INTENSITY STEADY-STATE TRAINING (LISS)<br>3 times a week | | | | | | | |
| STRENGTH<br>5 times a week<br>3 exercises—4 series of 20, 15, 12, and 10 repetitions<br>One day per group<br>Glutes—quadriceps—femorals—biceps/triceps—shoulders/back | | | | | | | |
| ABDOMINALS<br>3 days a week<br>3 exercises—4 series of 25 repetitions | | | | | | | |

Download https://www.fitplanapp.com/athletes/michelle-lewin, or train with my platform: www.lewinfitnessplatform.com.

# 12-WEEK PROGRESS CONTROL LOG

| MEASUREMENTS | 1 | | | 2 | | | | 3 | | | |
| --- | --- | --- | --- | --- | --- | --- | --- | --- | --- | --- | --- | --- |
| | WEEK 1 | WEEK 2 | WEEK 3 | WEEK 4 | WEEK 5 | WEEK 6 | WEEK 7 | WEEK 8 | WEEK 9 | WEEK 10 | WEEK 11 | WEEK 12 |
| NECK | | | | | | | | | | | | |
| CHEST | | | | | | | | | | | | |
| WAIST | | | | | | | | | | | | |
| HIPS | | | | | | | | | | | | |
| THIGHS | | | | | | | | | | | | |
| ARMS | | | | | | | | | | | | |
| WEIGHT | | | | | | | | | | | | |
| % BODY FAT | | | | | | | | | | | | |

# HEALTHY GROCERY LIST

Here is my grocery list of healthy ingredients, organized by proteins, fats, fresh vegetables, starches, legumes, whole grains, fruits, herbs and spices, dairy products, and other products.

## PROTEINS

- ☐ Chicken
- ☐ Turkey
- ☐ Pork tenderloin
- ☐ Eggs
- ☐ Meat (bison, beef tenderloin)
- ☐ Seafood and shellfish (prawns, shrimp, mussels, scallops, clams, lobster, squid, octopus)
- ☐ Bluefish, rich in omega-3 (fresh salmon, tuna, sardines, sea trout, mullet, eel, swordfish, lamprey)
- ☐ Whitefish (tilapia, grouper, mackerel, hake, bass, bonito, snapper, catfish, monkfish, anchovies, pout, cod, acedia, halibut, flounder, whiting, stingray, turbot)

## FATS

- ☐ Avocado
- ☐ Black olives
- ☐ Extra-virgin olive oil
- ☐ Olive or coconut oil spray
- ☐ Organic coconut oil
- ☐ Sesame oil
- ☐ Sesame seeds
- ☐ Almonds
- ☐ Hazelnuts
- ☐ Grated coconut (sugar-free)
- ☐ Tahini
- ☐ Flaxseeds
- ☐ Peanuts
- ☐ Cashews
- ☐ Nuts
- ☐ Pistachios

## FRESH VEGETABLES

- ☐ Chard
- ☐ Bell peppers
- ☐ Hot peppers (rocoto, habanero, jalapeño)
- ☐ Garlic
- ☐ Fresh basil
- ☐ Artichokes
- ☐ Leeks
- ☐ Eggplants
- ☐ Watercress
- ☐ Bok choy
- ☐ Broccoli
- ☐ Zucchini
- ☐ Water chestnuts
- ☐ Onions, green onions, or shallots
- ☐ White onions
- ☐ Purple or red onions
- ☐ Chives
- ☐ Celery
- ☐ Mushrooms
- ☐ Chayote
- ☐ Cilantro
- ☐ Brussels sprouts
- ☐ Cauliflower
- ☐ Asparagus
- ☐ Spinach
- ☐ Escarole
- ☐ Endive
- ☐ Fennel
- ☐ Ginger
- ☐ Jicama
- ☐ Kale
- ☐ Lettuce
- ☐ Romaine lettuce
- ☐ Lemongrass
- ☐ Chinese turnips
- ☐ Hearts of palm
- ☐ Cucumbers
- ☐ Parsley
- ☐ Chilies
- ☐ Red pepper
- ☐ Portobello mushrooms
- ☐ Japanese radish or daikon
- ☐ Cabbage
- ☐ Purple cabbage
- ☐ Radicchio
- ☐ Arugula
- ☐ Roma tomatoes
- ☐ Cherry tomatoes
- ☐ Sun-dried tomatoes or dehydrated tomatoes without oil

## VEGETABLES, TUBERS, AND STARCHY FRUITS

- ☐ Pumpkin
- ☐ Sweet potatoes or yams
- ☐ Potatoes
- ☐ Plantains
- ☐ Cassava or manioc
- ☐ Carrots

## LEGUMES

- ☐ Alfalfa
- ☐ Beans
- ☐ Chickpeas
- ☐ Peas
- ☐ Lentils
- ☐ Soy beans
- ☐ Green beans

## WHOLE GRAINS

- ☐ Brown rice (gluten-free)
- ☐ Rolled oats or oat bran
- ☐ Corn or cornmeal (gluten-free)
- ☐ Homemade popcorn (gluten-free)
- ☐ Quinoa (gluten-free)
- ☐ High-fiber whole wheat toast
- ☐ Brown rice crackers (gluten-free)

## FRUITS

- ☐ Blueberries
- ☐ Cherries
- ☐ Plums
- ☐ Peaches
- ☐ Strawberries
- ☐ Pomegranates
- ☐ Guavas
- ☐ Kiwis
- ☐ Lemons
- ☐ Limes
- ☐ Mandarins
- ☐ Natural green and red apples
- ☐ Mangoes
- ☐ Cantaloupes
- ☐ Peaches
- ☐ Blackberries
- ☐ Oranges
- ☐ Pears
- ☐ Pineapples
- ☐ Grapefruit
- ☐ Raisins

## HERBS AND SPICES

- ☐ Fresh basil
- ☐ Aniseed powder
- ☐ Saffron
- ☐ Cinnamon sticks and powder
- ☐ Cardamom
- ☐ Curry
- ☐ Chia seeds
- ☐ Chili powder
- ☐ Cloves
- ☐ Cumin
- ☐ Turmeric
- ☐ Dill
- ☐ Tarragon
- ☐ Hibiscus flowers
- ☐ Garam masala
- ☐ *Guayabita*

- ☐ Fresh peppermint
- ☐ Ginger
- ☐ Bay leaves
- ☐ Lemongrass
- ☐ Marjoram
- ☐ Nutmeg
- ☐ Oregano
- ☐ Paprika
- ☐ Peperoncino
- ☐ Black pepper
- ☐ Pink Himalayan sea salt
- ☐ Complete marinade seasoning
- ☐ All-Purpose Seasoning
- ☐ BBQ seasoning
- ☐ Five-spices flavoring
- ☐ Greek seasoning
- ☐ Thyme
- ☐ Rosemary
- ☐ Vanilla extract
- ☐ Za'atar

## DAIRY AND DAIRY PRODUCTS

- ☐ Greek yogurt (sugar-free)
- ☐ Cottage cheese (fat-free)

## MISCELLANEOUS

- ☐ Cocoa powder
- ☐ Instant coffee
- ☐ Dark sugar-free chocolate (70 percent)
- ☐ Natural stevia-based sweetener
- ☐ Light gelatin
- ☐ Grain mustard
- ☐ Tomato sauce (sodium-free)
- ☐ Traditional mustard, Dijon mustard, old-fashioned Dijon mustard
- ☐ Almond vegetarian cheese
- ☐ Ketchup (low sugar)
- ☐ Sriracha sauce
- ☐ Sugar-free maple syrup
- ☐ Green tea
- ☐ Black tea
- ☐ Balsamic vinegar
- ☐ Wine vinegar
- ☐ Apple cider vinegar
- ☐ Vanilla and chocolate whey protein

# ACKNOWLEDGMENTS

To my MOM, Sandra, for giving me life, unconditional love, protection, and the strength I needed to become who I am today.

To my SIBLINGS, Antonieta and Pascual, for sharing spaces of growth, joy, and dreams together and for being my engine to succeed in life.

To my GRANDMOTHER Ruth for being my greatest example of work, temperance, and strength.

To my husband and manager, JIMMY, for his love, protection, and unconditional support and for walking hand in hand with me on this path full of joys, discipline, and challenges.

To my friend SAMAR, doctor and coauthor of this book, for the fun moments we have shared over the past two years and for working so hard to find the scientific research that supports all my actions.

To my personal trainer, JUAN HERNÁNDEZ, for offering me all his commitment and experience to help me improve and take my body to a higher level during our workouts.

To my publisher, PENGUIN RANDOM HOUSE, for giving me the opportunity to fulfill this first dream in the United States and the world, in two languages.

To my literary agent, ALEYSO BRIDGER, for her guidance, effort, persistence, and patience to complete this editorial project.

To the PHOTOGRAPHY TEAM: Rubén Darío in photography; Liselotte Salinas in kitchen and food styling; Roberto Ramos in makeup; Antonio Delgado, our production assistant; and Eight Studio, the location for all the photos. Thank you for giving us your very best in order to achieve the magic of each photograph.

To the team of PROFESSIONALS OF HEALTH AND COMMUNICATIONS who worked with us to scientifically validate the entire contents of this book and helped me to express my messages and experiences: Audry Chacín (obesity doctor), Andrea Parra (clinical nutritionist), Carlos Lezama (sports nutritionist), Anna Paola Mannucci (cooking, and development of some recipes), and Tarek Yorde (writing and editing).

To MY COMMUNITY and all those who follow me, support me, and motivate me over social media every day.

THANK YOU!

# INDEX

Thai Chicken Vegetable Stir-Fry, 214–15
Turkey Stew + Mixed Salad with Avocado, 238
Vegetarian Cheese, Tomato, and Arugula
  Cauliflower Pizza, 228

Macro minerals, 50
Magnesium, 47, 50
Malodextrin, 38, 55
Manganese, 50
Marbled Fit Protein Cupcakes, 96
Mayonnaise, 56
Meats, 43, 56, 270, (see also Beef; Buffalo;
  Chicken; Pork; Turkey)
Meditation, 66
Memory loss, 29, 30
Menstruation, 66, 273
Menu substitutions, 244–51, 255
Menus (see Breakfast; Lunch; Dinner;
  Pre-workout snacks; Snacks)
Metabolism, 254
  basal metabolism, 33–34, 37
  determination of, 34
  diet and nutrition and, 35, 37–41
  exercise and, 36–37, 41
  revving up, 41
  slow, 35, 41
  vitamins and minerals and, 50
Mexican restaurants, 256–57
Micro minerals, 50
Middle Eastern restaurants, 257
Milk, 47, 56
Minerals, 48, 50, 54, 55, 260, 266
Monounsaturated fatty acids, 49
Mood swings, 29
Motivation, 11, 13–16, 18, 20, 69
Muffins:
  Egg Muffins + High-Fiber Whole Wheat
    Toast, 121
  Smoked Salmon Muffins + Sweet Potato and
    Beet Chips, 180–81
Muscle mass, 22, 24, 26, 29, 34, 50, 81
  supplements for increasing, 261–63
Mushrooms:
  Chicken-Stuffed Portobello Mushrooms +
    Pico de Gallo, 136
  Spinach Crepe Filled with Turkey and
    Mushrooms, 97–98
  Turkey and Mushroom Scrambled Eggs, 198
  Turkey Portobello Burger, 184–85

Non-starchy vegetables, 48
Nonessential amino acids, 43
Nuts, 44, 55, 56, 66, 117–18, 208

Oat bran, 55
Oatmeal:
  Chocolate Almond Oatmeal Drink, 115
  Oatmeal Arepa + Scrambled Eggs, 109–10
  Oatmeal Protein Cookies, 157
  Oatmeal Protein Drink with Strawberries, 92

Oatmeal Protein Waffles, 102
Oats, 55
Obesity, 21, 24
Olive oil, 30, 38, 55, 56, 269
Olives, 56
Omega-3 polyunsaturated fatty acids, 30, 43,
  44, 49, 56, 260, 266
Omega-6 polyunsaturated fatty acids, 49

Pancakes:
  Carrot Protein, 186–87
  Chocolate Protein, 107–8, 206
  Strawberry Protein, 111–12, 216
  Vanilla Cranberry Protein, 127
  Vanilla Protein, 154
Pancreas, 31, 45
Partially hydrogenated oils, 38
Peanut butter:
  Green Apple or Pear + Peanut Butter, 193, 243
  Peanut Butter Blondies, 147
  Peanut Butter Chocolate Protein Balls,
    113–14
  Peanut Butter Chocolate Protein Shakes, 101
Peas, 47
Pepper Steak + Baked Yucca Chips + Mixed
  Salad, 182–83
Peppers:
  Baked Eggs in Stuffed Peppers, 213
Peruvian restaurants, 256
Pesticides, 64
Phosphorus, 50
Phytates, 55
Phytochemicals, 48
Pico de Gallo:
  Chicken Chili Lettuce Wraps with, 220
  Chicken-Stuffed Portobello Mushrooms
    with, 136
  Crispy Fish Sticks + Baked Yucca Fries with,
    145–46
  Grilled Buffalo Ribeye with, 112–13
  Tuna Lettuce Wraps with, 199
Pineapple:
  Beef Tenderloin Kebabs + Baked Criollo
    Potatoes with Pineapple Coleslaw Salad,
    167–69
  Grilled Chicken and Sweet-and-Sour
    Mustard with Pineapple Coleslaw Salad,
    242–43
  Lemon Grilled Fish + Sweet Potato Puree
    with Pineapple Coleslaw Salad, 207
  Light Pineapple Gelatin, 208–9
  Pineapple Fit Protein Cupcake, 136
  Pineapple Shrimp Kebabs + Baked Sweet
    Potato + Green Salad, 103–4
  Pineapple Skin Infusion, 212, 217, 222, 227,
    232, 237, 241
Pistachio Fit Protein Cupcake, 165
Pizza:
  Egg and Vegetable Pizza + Sweet Potato
    Cubes, 200–1

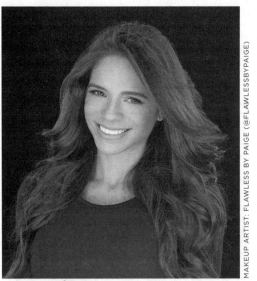

**MICHELLE LEWIN** is an internationally renowned fitness model. Born in Maracay, Venezuela, Lewin began training and modeling at an early age and later appeared in music videos and on magazine covers in her country. After competing in the NPC Bikini Competition, Lewin became one of the biggest stars in the fitness world. With a digital platform of more than 25 million followers, she is one of the most followed fitness gurus. Lewin lives with her husband, who is her manager and most important collaborator. She frequently participates as a fitness talent worldwide in countries such as India, Germany, Australia, Mexico, and Spain, and she has appeared on CNN, NBC, Telemundo, and in other international media.

## CONNECT ONLINE
michellelewin.com
facebook.com/FitnessMichelle

**Samar Yorde** is a Venezuelan doctor with a master's degree in health administration, obesity, and healthy living. She is a certified health coach in the United States, as well as an international speaker, writer, and author of three health-and-wellness books in Spanish. Dr. Yorde is the founder of *Soy Saludable*, a digital healthy-lifestyle platform on social media.